The Boy With the Wounded Thumb

The autobiographical account of the
world's leading innovator in veterinary
oncology and comparative cancer medicine

Gordon H. Theilen, DVM, ACVIM-Oncology

EDITPROS℮ SM

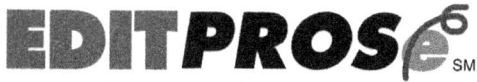

Published by EditPros LLC
423 F Street, Suite 206
Davis, CA 95616
www.editpros.com

ISBN: 978-1-937317-30-0

Library of Congress Control Number: 2017931780

Printed in the United States of America

CATALOGING INFORMATION:
Theilen, Gordon H.
The Boy With The Wounded Thumb

Filing Categories:

BIO019000   BIOGRAPHY & AUTOBIOGRAPHY / Educators

BIO017000   BIOGRAPHY & AUTOBIOGRAPHY / Medical

Dedication

I dedicate this book to initiators of new wisdom to benefit humans and animals.

Table of Contents

Foreword

By Richard B. Macfie, Captain, U.S. Navy (retired)

When Gordon invited me to write a foreword for this book, my first thought was the absurdity of a retired Navy captain (seagoing variety) trying to introduce the life work of a renowned researcher in the field of animal oncology. After some thought, it appeared to me that this book really tells two separate stories: one of my friend Gordon, and one of the professional accomplishments of Dr. Theilen. I will tackle the first and leave the second to Murray Gardner.

The Boy With the Wounded Thumb came into my life at Grant Elementary School in Richmond, California, in 1939. We embarked on a friendship that will last longer than we will. We went through grade and high schools together, were fraternity brothers at Cal, and Gordon was best man at my wedding. Since then, he and I have been mostly separated by geography and my naval career; but we have, nevertheless, proven that true friendship is affected by neither time nor space.

Gordon Theilen is the only man I have ever known who, as a little boy, knew to what he would dedicate his life – and then succeeded in fulfilling that dream. I have known some who did something because they (or someone) said they would – but were unhappy with the results.

Gordon not only followed his dream, but was eminently successful in his field and never lost the love he had for what he was doing.

Early in his practice as a veterinarian, he was frustrated by the frequency of cancers in animals and the absence of reference materials available for either diagnoses or treatments. In his search for answers, he found himself on a crusade that would envelop his professional life, take him around the world, and establish him as one of the world's foremost authorities on animal oncology. Despite his marvelous success in research, he always considered sharing his knowledge and findings with students a top priority.

Gordon was always a devout Christian and unalterably devoted to his wife Carolyn, their three children, grandchildren, and great grandchildren. They have weathered some tragic storms along the way. Carolyn fell victim to multiple sclerosis and has been severely disabled for many years. Then, their eldest son, Kyle, passed away while in his 50s. Their deep love for each other and for God has helped them weather each storm.

No book of or by Dr. Theilen would be complete without mention of his hobbies. In some of his free time, he has raised, bred, and trained Brittanys. He has also spent many years throughout the country as a field judge of hunting dogs. A few years ago, he was elected to the American Field Trial Hall of Fame.

Gordon invited me to write this foreword for *The Boy With the Wounded Thumb;* he did not ask me to write a book! I've tried to be brief, but find it difficult to say less about a man for whom I have such admiration and respect. I trust when you read his book the stone bond we have will be understandable.

Preface

This book is about much more than the severe thumb laceration that turned out to be a life-changing event for a 5-year-old boy. It is about what happened 22 years hence, when I obtained my degree in veterinary medicine. Even as I set out on a career as a young veterinary clinician, I could not foresee that I would follow a path into veterinary research that would lead me to participate in waging multidisciplinary "one medicine war" on cancer.

The mystery of cancer causation by retrovirus infection fascinated me, and I became continually determined to unlock the mysteries of why domesticated mammals develop forms of leukemia and sarcomas. Studies of stem cell sarcomas in turkeys, leukemia and sarcoma complex in cats, and simian leukemia and sarcoma complex provided enormous information on these cancers not only in animals, but also their oncogenes in humans. Control of retrovirus infection in cats and cattle led to control and prevention of leukemia. Colleagues and I discovered that ways to treat cancer using immunotherapy and prevention by vaccination were original ways to conquer cancer.

As a kid in rural Minnesota I did things out of the ordinary, climbing trees and creeping far out on branches looking for bird eggs, or scaling barn lofts to capture pigeons. My curiosity was ingrained. I conducted my first experiment at age 3, when I succeeded in seeing how a hen laid an egg. I hitched a team of horses to a wagon when I was 4, without parental supervision; I learned to swim without instruction. I learned to milk a cow at age 6, and I performed my first obstetrical veterinary procedure at 10 by correcting a breech delivery in a sow. At age 11 I began driving the first powered tractor my family owned.

School was an important priority. I walked two miles to a one-room school through the first five years of my education. As the sole student in my grade level, I progressed rapidly and excelled in a student body consisting of no more than 10 children from first through eighth grade. The gift of a sharp memory fostered my interest in history, geography, mathematics, and biology.

I was a kid who imagined great things when at play – usually alone. Creation through imagination with enjoyable toys made of rocks and wood was a necessity because store-bought toys were few and far between in my childhood. I played cowboys and Indians, galloping on a stick between my legs – a beautiful imaginary pinto, white or black stallion. That gift of imagination blossomed into creativity in the "one medicine war" on cancer.

I went beyond the expected to fulfill lifetime goals when stumbling blocks seemed impassable. I was guided and tempered by belief in Christ and strong relationships with my parents, sister, grandparents, other relatives, pastors, friends, colleagues, and students. Of great importance were the men and women of scientific status who carried me on their shoulders – as I describe in detail in *The Boy With the Wounded Thumb* and companion book *One Medicine War on Cancer*.

Acknowledgments

Writing *The Boy With the Wounded Thumb* was made possible with the assistance of Sacramento journalist Janet Fullwood, and the secretarial assistance of Melissa Wade of the Department of Surgical and Radiological Sciences in the School of Veterinary Medicine at the University of California, Davis.

Writing was inspired by my wife, Carolyn, family, friends, Dean Michael Lairmore and staff in the Office of the Dean at the UC Davis School of Veterinary Medicine. Pilar Rivera offered special encouragement and editorial advice. Marti Childs and Jeff March at EditPros in Davis, California, refined the manuscript and prepared the book for publication.

My parents, Ema and Lou Theilen, gave me freedom to develop individuality as a youngster and encouragement to pursue my educational goal of attaining a veterinary degree and becoming similarly gifted as Dr. R.F. Rasmussen, practitioner in 1930s Minnesota. All of my pastors and teachers, from Amy Anderson in first grade to high school and college, gave me the mental acumen to be original. Associations with Drs. Seymour Roberts and Robert Walker helped expose me to veterinary medicine as a high school and college student, and prepared me for what to anticipate in a lifelong career in veterinary medicine. I was blessed to be employed at the University of California, Davis, where I thrived on opportunities to be creative in the company of world-renowned scientists, leading to the establishment of the discipline of veterinary oncology through which to wage war on cancer.

CHAPTER 1

Minnesota, Where It All Began

"You can observe a lot just watching."
– Yogi Berra

I was born at the end of the Roaring Twenties, and the Great Depression enveloped most of my childhood years. I was a jaundiced newborn, yellow as a banana, for the first month after my birth on May 29, 1928. I mostly suckled and slept. Women in those days were required to stay in bed in the hospital for seven days after giving birth, so my first week of life was spent in the Montevideo, Minnesota, hospital.

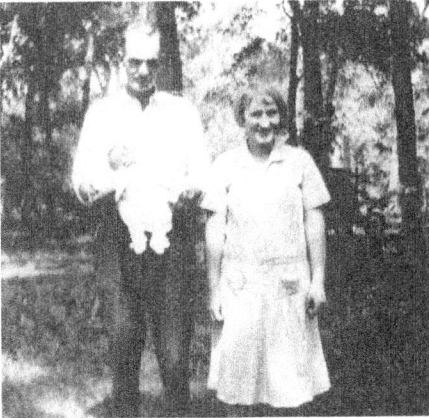

My Dad holding me, standing by Mom on Baptismal day, 34 days after my birth.

I was the first-born and only son of Ema Kathryn (née Schaller) Theilen, 22, and Ludwig (affectionately called "Lou") Theilen, 27. On Sunday, July 1, at 11:15 a.m., I was baptized Gordon Henry Theilen by Pastor H.W. Meohring of St. Paul's Lutheran Church. Pastor Meohring's sister made my white baptismal garments.

1

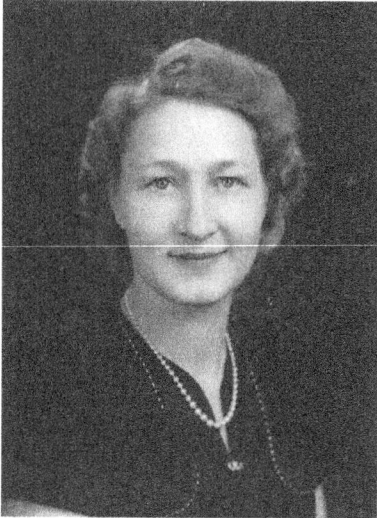

My mother, Ema

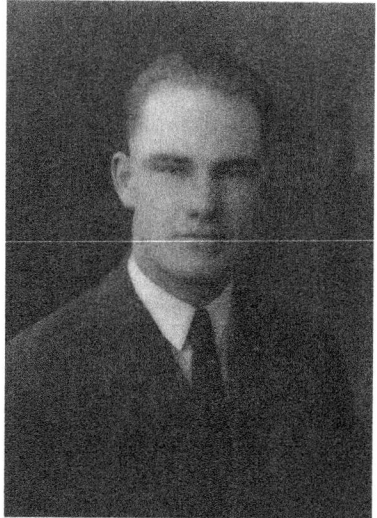

My father, Lou

My baptismal sponsors were my grandfather Henry Schaller and my aunt Margarie "Sidy" Theilen, who was 17 years old at the time. Margarie's son and daughter-in-law, James and Rae Nanaga of Fort Dodge, Iowa, told me that during Margarie's last years on Earth, well into her 90s when she was suffering the malady of Alzheimer's disease, she still remembered being my baptismal sponsor.

Being a sponsor was an awesome responsibility in the Lutheran church centuries before and even into the 1920s. Sponsors were requested to insure Christian upbringing; if parents should die the sponsors often became foster parents. Baptismal certificates were prepared as official documents because they represented an individual's identity, and were used as birth certificates for children born at home.

Aunt Gertie, who was Grandma Theilen's daughter, and her younger sister, Sidy, would come to Minnesota from Iowa, a distance of 200 miles. They often would hitchhike – not dangerous in those days of the early to mid-1930s. I always had a close relationship with Sidy. When Gertie and Sidy were ready to return home, they usually could not find their shoes. I had hidden their shoes because I did not want them to leave. The closest neighbors with a boy my age lived two miles from our house, and I longed for visits by aunts, other relatives, and friends to lessen loneliness and boredom of being alone.

1928 to 1932

The area around Montevideo is mostly flat, agriculturally developed prairie, as level as the Sacramento Valley in California where I later would live. Field corn and soybeans were the main crops, but other grains including wheat, barley, flax, and buckwheat were grown.

We lived on the Behren farm during the years after my birth until I reached the age of 4. The farm was on a county road about three miles north and one mile west of Montevideo, a half-mile east of the Chippewa River. The river wound through a gorge 100 feet below the surrounding farmland. On the eastern side of the river ran the Great Northern Railway, built sometime around the 1880s. Train whistles were loud and extremely piercing on cold winter nights, when sound carried at a higher pitch than on warm days.

May 29 always was a happy date in my young life, as mother and grandmother never forgot to hold a birthday party for me, albeit small in number of attendees and with few amenities. Grandma Schaller always baked an angel-food cake, which became my favorite. In later years, I learned that I shared my birth date with people of international acclaim, including Bob Hope, Shirley Temple, and President Jack Kennedy. Several good friends also had a May 29 birth date, including Ursula Straub, the wife of Otto Straub, a veterinary medicine friend in Tübingen, Germany.

From Ice Age to present

The eastern half of the former Territory of Minnesota, the "Land of 10,000 Lakes," became the state of Minnesota, the nation's 32nd state, on May 11, 1858. In the last Ice Age, 10,000 years ago, Minnesota was covered in ice. As the ice receded, glacial moraines carved out deep craters that filled with water to become lakes. The largest were Lake of the Woods near the town of Warroad, and Lake Superior, largest of the five Great Lakes, bordering on Canada.

The Anishinaabe, a group of indigenous people related to the Mdewakanton Band of the Dakota Nation, inhabited most of Minnesota for several centuries before Europeans. Spanish explorers arrived in 1650, having probed their way up the Mississippi River from Louisiana's Gulf Coast. On an early exploration, the explorers traveled westward along the Minnesota River, which empties into the Mississippi River near present-day Minneapolis. Their path led them about 130 miles upstream to the present town of Granite Falls, and then 14 miles north to a spot atop the bluffs that they named Montevideo. Translated from Spanish "monte" (mountain) and "vista" (view), the name often is loosely translated as "I see a mountain."

This was where the "Boy With the Wounded Thumb" was born approximately 278 years later, and 78 years after the first Christian missionaries brought the Triune God to the area and established a mission outpost at Lac qui Parle (the "lake that speaks," a translation from Dakota Sioux), 30 miles north of Montevideo.

Settlers enticed by the federal Homestead Act, which granted 160 acres of undeveloped land to any man or woman 21 years old or the head of a family, came to the area in the 1870s. The first Lutheran missionary pastors in the area arrived at the same time. The Catholic priests who followed the Spanish explorers initiated Christianity in the mid-1800s. Minnesota evolved to become the most Lutheran state in the country, with Lutherans constituting 23 percent of the state's population by the turn of the 21st century. People of Scandinavian and German background accounted for the heavy influx of the Lutheran denomination.

Minnesota is the country's twelfth-largest state in terms of geographic area. It is known for moderation in politics and is ethnically dominated by people of Scandinavian and northern European heritage. However, a large number of Hispanic agricultural workers are seasonally present, along with people of other ethnicities. For instance, the first Muslim elected to the House of Representatives is from Minnesota. Keith Ellison was sworn in and took his oath not by placing his hand on the Holy Christian Bible, but rather on the Koran. His election likely was facilitated due to liberalization of thought in politics and religion – progressive or liberation theology and politics.

Minnesota's Scandinavian heritage

Minnesotans whose ancestors spoke Northern European Germanic languages have a noticeable accent and a special, Scandinavian type of humor quite different from the humor of the Eastern part of the United States, which is derived to a large extent from Jewish heritage. You betcha.

Garrison Keillor, whose *A Prairie Home Companion* variety radio program was broadcast from the Twin Cities (Minneapolis and St. Paul), did much to popularize the Scandinavian humor of Minnesota, the Dakotas, and Wisconsin. I remember examples of this type of humor from an early age – hearing Norwegians, for example, needling Swedish persons by saying "Ten thousand Sveeds chased thru de veeds by vone Norvegian."

Swedish and Norwegian immigrants had not forgotten Norway's declaration of independence from Sweden in the 1800s and the military battles that occurred before Norway was granted independence. By contrast, we Americans can identify our independence from Great Britain and a new uniquely written national Constitution.

Minnesotans experience dramatic changes in weather, especially along the state's northern and western borders. I remember walking to school in temperatures well below zero degrees Fahrenheit. Summer temperatures in the Montevideo area can exceed 100 degrees in July and August. Tornadoes are a frequently encountered annoyance from May through August, but they generally are less severe than twisters that occur in Texas and the Central Plains states.

5

CHAPTER 2

Depression and Poverty

"I have found out in later years that we were very poor,
but the glory of America is that we didn't know it then."
– Dwight D. Eisenhower

Most farm families were poor, including the Lou Theilen family, along with millions of others. In the 1920s, the Dwight Eisenhower family from Kansas was among those who lived a life of austerity. A severe drought wracked the middle of the nation in the 1930s "Dust Bowl." Large numbers of farms with loans were foreclosed by banks, insurance companies and other corporate investors. Crop failures and depressed prices for farm produce sped sharecrop farmers to sell possessions and resulted in a mass exodus from rural to city living. My parents began married life as sharecoppers in 1926 and never owned farm land. Sharecoppers were so called because a percentage of their crop income paid the lease. They lived on three different farms owned by insurance companies, and in 1939 lived with great uncle and aunt Theilen in anticipation of becoming owners. That did not materialize, leading to our family's eventual move west.

The drought took its greatest toll on farm-family populations of Wisconsin, Minnesota, North and South Dakota, Nebraska, Kansas, Colorado, Oklahoma, Arkansas, and Texas, but all farm communities throughout the nation were affected. However, the most sweeping changes took place in the rural way of life in the Midwest.

Until that period in history, small family farms of 80 to 120 acres had been sufficient in size to generate enough income to support a family with several children. Vegetable gardens could be found on every farm, as families raised ample amounts and varieties for canning in glass jars for winter subsistence. Enough animals were butchered to maintain a meat supply for a large family during the winter months. Bacon, ham, and sausages were cured in a smokehouse and hung in the cellar. Most farm women raised chickens, geese, and ducks to help support family income. Sales provided enough money to keep the family stocked with purchased staples such as salt, sugar, and clothing not easily made at home.

Farms in the Midwest produced numerous types of crops and had a variety of livestock. Crops such as oats, wheat, rye, and field corn were grown primarily to feed animals. Most farms counted dairy and beef cattle, hogs, draft horses, chickens, ducks, and geese among their menageries. Upper Midwest farms usually did not raise sheep or goats; we had some sheep on our farm during the last year there.

After World War II, the average size of farms increased substantially in order to remain sustainable. Farming became much less diversified, as growers began to specialize in specific types of agriculture, such as strictly row crops, or growing wheat exclusively, or raising only one species of livestock, such as pigs or cattle, and so forth.

These changes, brought on by drought and economic depression, eventually induced the Theilen family to migrate to California in 1939. Our story was similar to that of migrant farm families that John Steinbeck portrayed in his book *The Grapes of Wrath.*

Our family was on the move, motivated by hopes of my father finding work somewhere in the West, as he fully believed he would. It is hard to imagine that a family of four with a net worth of $1,000 would wander with the intention of resettling 2,000 or more miles away from friends and relatives. We were part of a mass migration from farm living to city dwelling. Even on the journey I really missed the myriad things that used to occupy my time as a rural dweller.

Love for animals

My constant companion until I was 10 was a purebred German shepherd dog, "Rex," who was related to Playfellows, seen in the movies of the late 1920s. I enjoyed the companionship of sitting on Dad's draft horses and pretending to ride a fine saddle horse. No longer was there a need to pretend that a stick between my legs was a horse. I always wanted a pony of my own, and draft horses were the closest we had to a saddle horse.

Forty years later I purchased my first real saddle horse, Sunday, a 15-year-old mare, from a colleague, John Hughes, DVM. Sunday was a large-boned gray-and-white mare who probably had some draft-horse blood in her pedigree. This was somewhat ironic, as the only riding horses I'd experienced up until this time were Dad's draft horses, which I was allowed to ride only when they were not needed for work.

I remember riding bareback with bridle only, dressed in coveralls, without a shirt and with my feet bare. Going away from the farm, the horse would walk along very slowly. But when turned for home, it would canter with eagerness – and, sure enough, I would bounce off and have to walk the rest of the way home. Nevertheless, when given the chance, I would ride the next available

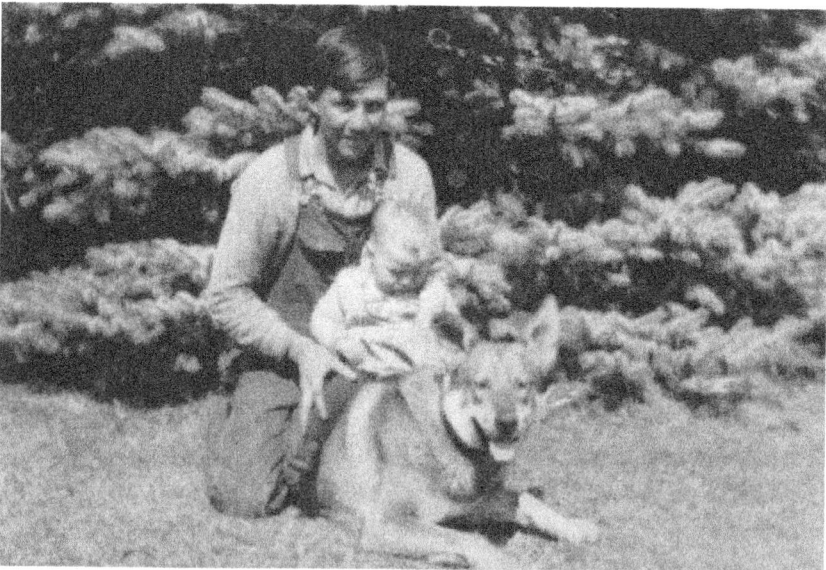

Our purebred German shepherd dog, Rex, a friend and me, age 4 months.

draft horse again, with the same results. Luckily, I never was injured beyond a few bruises and skin abrasions.

I rode only during summer vacation time, and always in bare feet with no saddle, only a bridle with reins. The horse would know automatically to go back to its assigned stall in the barn. Later in life, I experienced several horse accidents, but my infatuation with horses (and a mule) did not cease. As most equestrians know from experience, there is no such thing as a safe horse. I always wondered how the Indians of the Western plains could so successfully ride a galloping horse at full speed, bareback and with nothing more than a reed bridle with hand-woven reins.

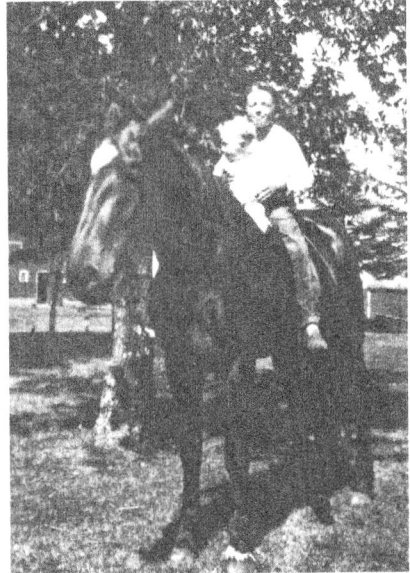

Draft horse mare Molly, Eddie Schaeffer, and me at 12 months old.

When I was 4 years old, we moved east about eight miles to the Thompson farm. My oldest memories of childhood experiences began there. That's where I began to develop understanding of the trials and tribulations of sharecrop farming in western Minnesota during the drought-stricken years of the Depression.

During a period of 12 years, I lived on four different farms, all but one purchased by insurance companies following the Wall Street crash of 1929. We were a close family during those difficult times. My Dad was the finest man I knew and would ever know. He lived a life closest to that of being a "little Christ," as perfect as one can be following Jesus.

These early years were filled with memories of childhood experiences and the difficult economic times the family had experienced. This early childhood history blended with memories of experiences beginning at age 5 with expanding clarity after I entered first grade in a one-room country school at 6 years of age.

My Molly mule, Derby. I'm holding Field Champion Jean-Luc Le Breton.

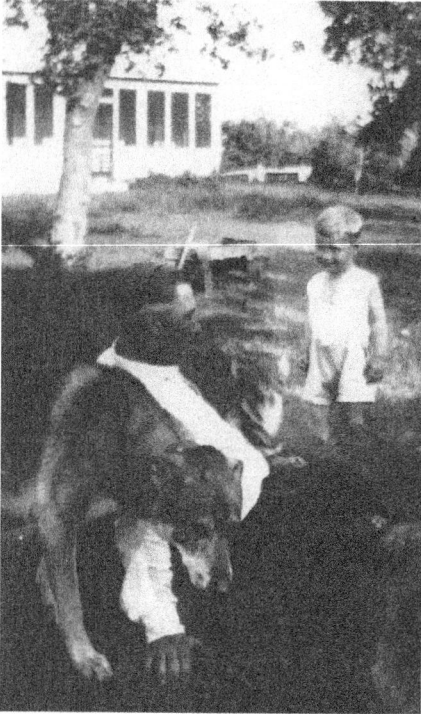

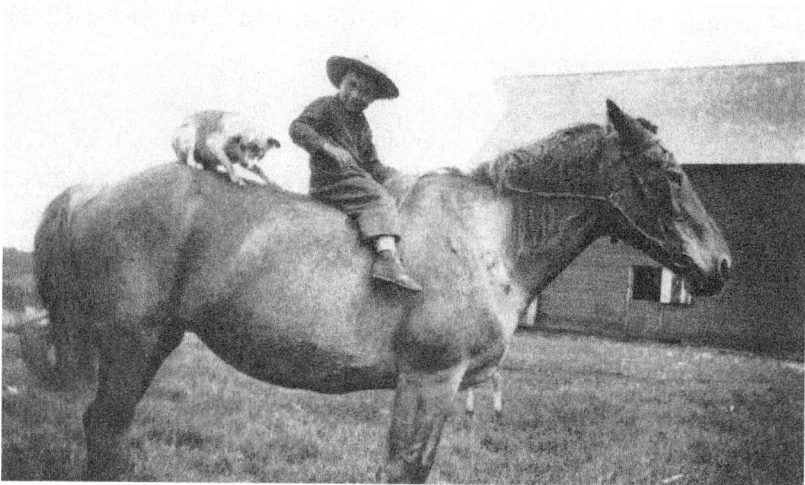

Uncle Charlie playing with Rex, when I was 18 months old.

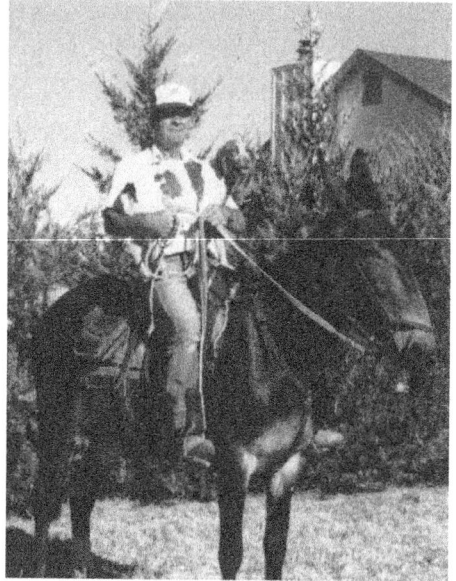

Draft horse mare Molly, my terrier-type dog Tricksy, and me at age 5.

CHAPTER 3

A Life-Changing Event at 5 Years of Age

"On such small points of agates does the world revolve."
– Winston Churchill

Wounded thumb

I became interested in veterinary medicine as a 5-year-old, when a horrific accident occurred. I wanted to help my mother split kindling needed to start the wood range-stove in preparation for the noon meal. Five-year-olds usually are in the way and want to help mom.

On our Minnesota farm, the primary meal of the day was "dinner," not lunch. Dr. R.F. Rasmussen. DVM, was vaccinating pigs for hog cholera on the farm that day. All present when mealtime rolled around were invited to eat with the family. In those days, there were no fast-food restaurants. Minnesota hospitality was the mode for every day.

I wanted Mom to chop a piece of wood I was holding, and she did not hesitate to swing the hand held hatchet. "Gordon, step back," she said as the blade came down. As it did, I quickly slipped into the path of the ax with the wood I held in my right hand. In the blink of an eye, my right thumb was nearly severed from the first to the second phalanx, cutting right through the joint. Blood spurted from the wound. I don't remember crying; that was a trait

11

I rarely resorted to when injured because I was raised with the credo that "men do not cry."

Mom urgently hollered to Dad, who was helping Dr. Rasmussen in the pig barn, to please come to the house immediately. "Gordon has a severe injury of his hand." The two men stopped what they were doing and hurriedly ran to the house. Blood was plentifully on my right hand and clothing.

Dr. Rasmussen calmly and carefully cleaned the traumatized thumb with dilute Lysol solution before applying a tourniquet at the base of the thumb until major hemorrhage ceased. After cleaning the severe laceration, Dr. Rasmussen applied pressure and completely wrapped my thumb in a gauze bandage. He did not suture the wound, but applied a splint, and instructed me to keep the bandage dry. The splint was removed five days later, with no evidence of wound dehiscence (rupturing). I maintained full use of the thumb once it healed, but a permanent scar reminded me of that fateful occurrence every day afterward.

Dr. Rasmussen took an interest in me, and he became my hero. From that point onward, I never wavered from wanting to become a veterinarian. The accident turned out to be a huge blessing. Twenty-two years later, when I graduated from veterinary school with a DVM diploma held in my scarred right hand, I had an unsurpassed feeling of fulfillment.

My parents gracefully accepted Dr. Rasmussen's gratis and efficient fix of the wounded thumb as highly adequate medical attention. Dr. Rasmussen, who had graduated from Iowa State with a DVM degree in 1931, was a capable veterinarian who efficiently practiced "one medicine," frequently done in those days.

A trip to "Monte" (Montevideo) to see the town medical doctor by the name of Rous was not necessary, and anyhow it would have cost a dozen eggs, a quart of fresh milk, and some vegetables. Bartering was a way of life, and often farmers would obtain staples such as flour and sugar at the Monte grocery store in exchange for eggs and milk from their farms. In the 21st century, a person without means to pay for medical help can go straight to the emergency room and obtain medical treatment. But on a drought-sickened Minnesota farm in the 1930s, that wasn't an option.

As a child, I always was available to help when an animal needed doctoring. At age 6, I milked a cow assigned to me and helped in small ways in watering and feeding calves, barn cats, and other animals. Animals were part of the economic unit of versatile Minnesota farming; the barn cats kept the rodent population at bay. Young kids were part of the labor force needed to help run the farm.

The thumb accident changed my life forever and set in motion, 18 years later, the commencement of an education in veterinary medicine. I was the first to be given the opportunity to initiate the specialty of veterinary cancer medicine, and was among a few internationally known veterinarians at the time who appreciated the need for a new discipline – as I'll explain in greater detail in my associated book *One Medicine War on Cancer*.

As a veterinarian, I had opportunities to discover viruses that caused cancer, and to explore the realm of cells that become cancerous. I was among a group of pioneers who isolated and studied a group of retroviruses (RNA tumor viruses) that caused cancer, especially leukemia, lymphoma, and sarcoma, in a variety of domesticated animal and primate species.

Austere living conditions

Life on a farm in Minnesota in the early 1930s was far from convenient. Lighting was by kerosene lamps or pressurized white-gas lanterns. Heating was by pot-bellied stoves and the wood cook-stove that produced heat by burning mostly corn cobs or chopped wood. Coal was too expensive for most sharecropper families to afford.

Wintertime was cold even in the house. Storm windows were installed each October, but even then, the inside pane would ice over. Water had to be carried in, and stood in a three- to five-gallon bucket on a counter near the cook-stove. We had no running water or plumbing. Adults used outside toilets. Corn cobs or Sears and Montgomery Ward catalog pages served as toilet paper. In winter, snow sprinkled the toilet seats. A common expression used in reference to cleaning oneself after defecation was "cold as a cob."

Children used a bucket for toilet needs. Food scraps also went in the bucket, which was referred to as a "slop or swill bucket" and was taken each day to the pig barn for adding to the porcine diet.

Clothes were hand-washed using a washboard sitting in a 10-gallon, galvanized tub. Clothing also was rinsed by hand, then dried outdoors on a clothesline. In wintertime, the wash was brought into the house frozen, then thawed and dried on hampers arrayed around the pot-bellied stove.

Farm families made laundry soap by boiling tallow and lye, which gelled when cooled. They usually purchased hand and bath soap. Bathing customarily was done on Saturday nights in the same 10-gallon, galvanized tub that served as a laundry basin. The rest of the week, bodies were hand-washed with washcloths. Men shaved with a straight-blade razor sharpened on a smooth leather strop that hung near a mirror in the kitchen.

Radio was a new means of communication during my childhood. Radio receivers were powered by batteries, and some homes had wind-driven generators for charging batteries. Most kids were allowed to listen to radio programs after school in the wintertime at around 5 or 6 p.m. *Little Orphan Annie, Renfrew of the Royal Mounted,* and *The Lone Ranger* were favorite children's programs. Wintertime darkness would come around at 4 p.m. and daybreak at 8:30 a.m.

Iodine and Lysol were the commonly used antiseptics, while gauze and adhesive tape were available for purchase for covering wounds. Salves were commonly used. One of the most popular, Bag Balm, first made in 1899 by Dairy Association Company in Lyndonville, Vermont, was used to treat sores on cows' teats and udders. Of all the products found around the house in my growing-up years, the only one still used by our family on sores is Bag Balm. It is a thick, yellowish salve with a strong medicinal odor that lasts for several minutes when applied on chronic, non-healing wounds.

Men and some women chewed tobacco, used snuff, or rolled their own cigarettes. Men often smoked pipes, customarily, Prince Albert tobacco in a red can. Kids smoked dried cornsilk, rolled with cigarette papers taken secretly from an adult's stash.

Crank telephones

Alexander Graham Bell's invention was present on most farms as early as the mid-1920s. Most were connected with party lines that served six to ten farms. To use the telephone we would lift the receiver earpiece from the hanger and then crank the handle clockwise to signal the local operator that we wanted to make a phone call. She would say, for example, "Gordon, what number do you want to reach?"

I had the privilege of calling my Grandmother Schaller, and would tell the operator, "10-B-25, please." It's amazing that I can still remember my grandparents' telephone number after not using it for six and a half decades!

There were always those among the farm families sharing the line who would listen in to learn what their neighbors were up to. We called them "rubber necks." Telephone operators had fantastic memories and could recognize all the callers within their area. While I lived on the Thompson farm the operator was based in Maynard, the nearest town.

My sister's birth

I was an only child for five and a half years until my sister, Blythe, my only sibling, was born on November 16, 1933, while we lived on the Thompson farm. It was unseasonably cold, and a substantial blizzard had produced deep snow.

I clearly remember my sixth birthday party. As the small group awaited lifelong friend Lloyd Menking's return home from school, Mom said to his mother, Trena, "Gordon will go to school next year." That sent a thrill up my spine that I distinctly recall 82 years later.

Birthday parties involved a cake. Grandmother Schaller baked an angel food cake made with the whites of a dozen eggs. The frosting was homemade. We also had ice cream, hand-churned with ice purchased at the local ice house. The ice house, very well insulated, was layered six or more feet high with 30-pound blocks of ice separated by layers of sawdust to keep them from sticking together when the weather warmed. Ice cream was made by adding salt to ice during churning, which created a cold brine that lowered the temperature to below zero – necessary to freeze cream ingredients. In the winter, ice was everywhere.

First grade, fall 1934 – and reverie 78 years later

I started country school in the fall of 1934, attending a schoolhouse about a mile west of the Thompson farm. My teacher from first grade through most of third grade was Miss Amy Anderson. She is the only country-school teacher whose name I remember, and I was hoping to visit her in July 1999 when I attended a Schaller family reunion in Maynard.

I asked while visiting with Lloyd Menking in 1999 if he knew where Amy Anderson lived. He indicated she had lived in Benson, Minnesota, about 10 miles north of Monte. Lloyd found out through inquiries that Amy had died a few months earlier. It would have been a wonderful experience for me to see her again after 63 years, and for her to learn that one of her students had gone on to become a veterinarian and university professor who devoted an entire career to teaching and cancer research. She most assuredly would have liked to know about her students' destinies. As a teacher, I always liked to learn about the accomplishments of former students and their lives after graduation.

On June 30, 2011, I was in a hospital room with my wife, Carolyn, who had suffered a concussion from a fall. The chaplain at Woodland Memorial Hospital came into her room. She wondered if we needed spiritual care, and the answer was yes. Our pastor, the Rev. Scott Stone, had been in the day before and held prayer and a Bible reading from Psalm 46, which Luther expanded upon, and which inspired him to write the famous Reformation hymn, "A Mighty Fortress Is Our God."

The devotion was consummated by saying the Lord's Prayer. As the words were being recited by those in attendance (our "adopted" family member Mari-Ann, her son, Kevin Green, Pastor Stone, Carolyn, and me), Carolyn came out of the coma and clearly repeated the words in unison with the rest of us. The chaplain, Dr. Donna Waterman, DVM, was impressed that Carolyn had briefly become cognitive while still in a coma.

I learned that Donna was a former veterinary student of mine who had changed professions several years previously. I did not recognize her. However, another friend, Mary Cullor, who was hospitalized on the same floor as Carolyn, said to me, "Did you know that Donna Waterman was one of your former students?" I hadn't realized that. But upon learning that, I had Donna paged to come to room 302A.

"Why did you not indicate you were one of my former students?" I asked. She replied that she was embarrassed to indicate that she became a chaplain, because she thought it would have been a disappointment to me that she left veterinary medicine for a different profession.

I was reading a book at the time about John Wooden, the famous UCLA basketball coach, who was a devout Christian. He discussed the seven guiding principles that his father had given him when he graduated from the eighth grade. I discussed with Donna the concept of the "balanced triad," which I had passed on to my students as a guide to leading a successful life as a veterinarian. (See chapter 14 for more on a balanced triad, an axiom to a successful professional life.) I then indicated to Donna that I believed the highest calling in life was the Christian ministry.

This brought a smile upon Donna's face, and she gave me a hug before leaving the room. It was the day of her retirement as a chaplain. What a coincidence to have had such a wonderful meeting with a former student and to learn the story of her life. This made my day and week, despite the fact that, at the same time, Carolyn was recovering from a nasty concussion and in a coma.

First to third grades

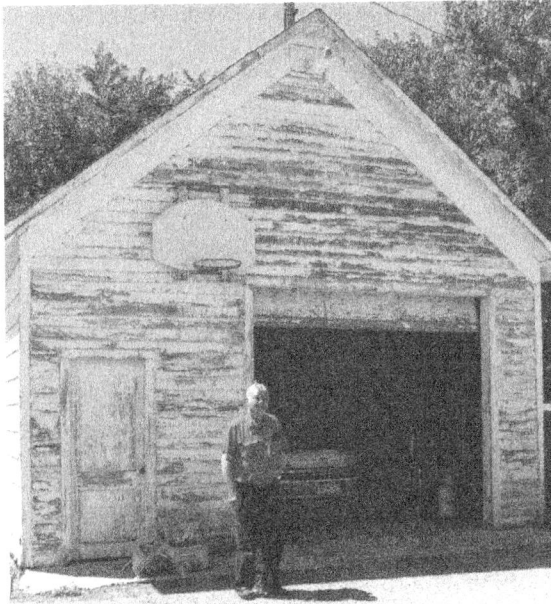

Me standing alongside the former one-room school district 23 building, which my cousin Odell Schaller purchased from the school district and now uses as a shop and garage.

From my first to third year in grade school, I attended Leenthrop Township School District 23 in Chippewa County. It consisted of a single sturdy white building. That one-room building had a rear entrance that led through a coat and mud-boot room to the classroom. Four rows each containing five desks faced the teacher's desk in front, next to the wood-and-coal-burning stove.

In 2001, my cousin Odell Schaller purchased the building from Leenthrop

Township. It now stands on his farm, three miles south of its location when I attended classes 65 years earlier. Coincidences of many types have happened continuously in my lifetime. Nothing, I have learned, happens by chance.

Scholastic achievements

In the 1930s, if students did not pass state requirements for moving on to the next grade, they repeated the grade. It seems almost unimaginable now, but many never advanced beyond the fourth, sixth, or eighth grade. I progressed on my own scholastic pace. Few parents were interested in their children going beyond eighth grade, and only exceptional students went to high school. Of my Minnesota school friends through the fifth grade, none sought college degrees, nor did any of my Minnesota relatives.

My sister, Blythe, and I were among few from those poor Minnesota farm families who sought to continue beyond eighth grade. We were fortunate to have parents who encouraged higher education. The wounded thumb accident had motivated me since age 5 to continue school to become a veterinarian.

Polydactylism: extra digits in man and beast

Children from one family at our school had an anomaly known as polydactylia – more than five fingers on a hand, some fused together. I do not remember seeing their toes, which also might have been fused. Their parents were cousins of each other. Due to a close genetic relationship, complicated by low IQs, they inherited polydactylism. Penalties of intermarrying were obvious in this family. Two of the affected brothers had been in the eighth grade for a few years and would play with the younger kids and enjoyed their games as if they were younger than their real age. Polydactylism may be associated with shortened limbs in the offspring of afflicted parents. This is a genetic problem in a family acquaintance of a woman who married a man with webbed toes.

The family had three children: a daughter and two sons. The daughter and a son had short defective arms and polydactylia of the fingers. The daughter married a man with normal limbs. They in turn had a daughter and two sons. One son and the daughter had shortened arms with polydactylia. Their daughter (third generation) married a man with normal limbs, and the resulting son had drastically shortened arms. Children's limbs in this family became shorter with succeeding generations and seemed to demonstrate that polydactylism is a dominant inherited trait, with severity increased in succeeding generations.

I had encountered polydactylism as a first-grader and again later in veterinary medicine, where I learned at an international genetic conference that dogs with webbed toes also gave birth to offspring with shortened limbs. Shortened limbs in newborn children in the 1970s were associated with mothers taking thalidomide, a tranquilizer, during the first trimester of pregnancy. The memory of Polydactylism is an indication of my interest in medical conditions found in both humans and animals at an early age

CHAPTER 4

Other Boyhood Memories

"You will find a joy in overcoming obstacles."

– Helen Keller

Poor judgment

One day, walking home from school along the township road in late April 1935, after the snow had melted, I placed my metal lunch bucket in a deep drainage ditch full of water, and it floated away.

This was a valuable object and I wanted to retrieve it; however, I did not know how to swim. I went into the water chest-deep, and in so doing hit a rock with my left knee and sustained a deep laceration resulting in a scar that I still carry, alongside a scar from total knee replacement surgery performed on May 14, 2007. Knee replacement surgery gave me, while recuperating, an opportunity to began writing *The Boy With the Wounded Thumb*.

After I climbed out of that drainage ditch, my father came along while grading the gravel road with a team of horses and found me soaking wet. He gave me an emotional lecture about the dangers of drowning, impressing upon me that losing a lunch bucket was not so important. From my point of view, I was just being a boy who wanted to experiment with a lunch bucket being a boat. I clearly remember Dad's gentleness despite my poor judgment.

That was my juvenile personality: go to the limit in everyday experiences and don't be bothered with the consequences. I have often stated that my Dad was the finest man I ever knew. He lived a life of Christian principles, concerned about others and always ready to help those in need. His presence was comforting.

The last time I saw Dad was on a March day in 1964 during a short visit to California for research matters at the University of California, Davis. I was doing a fellowship at the National Cancer Center, part of the National Institutes of Health in Bethesda, Maryland. Dad did not go to work until I left at about 8 a.m. to catch a plane from San Francisco to Dulles Airport in Virginia. As I drove away, looking back, I saw Dad had a worried, strained, and sad expression on his face, as though he wanted to say more before I departed. I felt and anticipated at the moment I drove away that we would not see each other again in this life. In less than a month, Dad died of a massive heart attack.

The world revolves on such small moments of intuition. I have experienced them often when saying goodbyes to loved ones, including my grandparents, friends, and other relatives. The experience of saying last goodbyes is lengthy and gets longer with advancing age. Many wonderful relatives, friends, former students, and colleagues have died as I live on.

1935–1936: Memories of a Model T

I was expected to walk to school, during rain, snow, sleet, or sunshine. On many days, Mr. Olaf Nelson would pick up the Menking boys, Lloyd and Francis, as they walked from their farm lane. I was usually walking along further on from the Menking farm, and Olaf would stop his Model T Ford touring car and ask, "Gordon, do you want a ride?"

Olaf always drove Ellis, his only child, three miles to school. It was known that Ellis was spoiled. Interestingly, Olaf would always be chewing tobacco, and spit down the steering column, aiming for holes in the floorboards. He would not spit out the side of the touring Model T, as spit would fly right back into the open-sided car and hit passengers in the back seat. The steering column was inches thick with dried and freshly spit tobacco juice. Ellis became an alcoholic and died at an early age from liver cirrhosis. Lloyd, Francis, and I lived on into eight decades of life and remembered those rides to school.

21

A fascination with pigeons

I was an avid admirer of birds and curious about the various egg colors. Pigeons were a challenge to catch. I caught most of them in barn cupolas by crawling hand-over-hand along metal hay carriers, with my feet dangling over the haymow floor. Once I was within range, the rest was easy. Pigeons sitting on nests would not move until I was inside the cupola, blocking their exit. Upon catching a pigeon, I crossed their wings, locking them in place so they could not fly, and dropped them safely onto hay below. I must have temporarily cleared pigeons from every farmer's barn for few miles within bicycling distance of our farm.

As an octogenarian now, I maintain a pigeon colony. The birds are trained to crawl through an open cone in order to re-enter the pen. These pigeons are used in bird dog training, as natural homers. When released they will fly back to the pen a distance of several miles. Pigeons are interesting birds and can serve as semi-pets.

Pigeons mate for life, but if a mate dies, the survivor may mate again. Both members of the pair sit on a nest containing two eggs, which hatch in 21 days. The newly hatched are known as squabs. Eyes open five or six days after hatching. Squabs are covered in downy feathers light to white in color.

Within two weeks after hatching, they show aggression by puffing themselves up to appear as if they are much larger birds. Their long beaks give them a dinosaur-like appearance. Some 110 million years ago, flying dinosaurs known as pterosaurs inhabited the Earth. Many such species of flying dinosaurs have been identified. Recently, a link between several species of pterosaurs has been found from England to China and Brazil. Pigeons, too, are found worldwide.

The young birds change appearance at about two months of age and began to look pigeon-like. They fly at this early age, being fully feathered. Feral pigeons are a light blue-gray with banding of black streaks in wings and body. Domesticated pigeons have colors from gray-blue to solid white or spotting of white and other colors. In birds that are solid blue-gray, the breast portion of the body, known as the crop, has an iridescent glow when seen in sunlight. It is an amazing phenomenon that gives the appearance of sun reflecting off water or snow crystals.

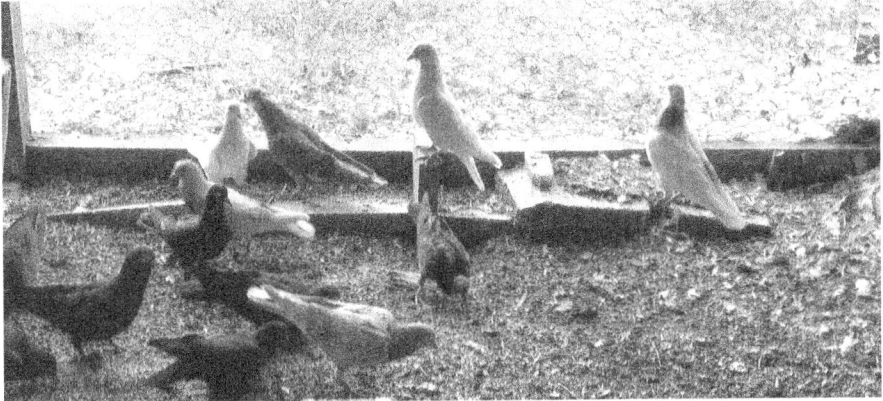

Pigeons in my pen in 2016. Pigeons are special birds that played a role in my boyhood development and personality (Photo by Christine Ortego).

To show dominance, birds walk up to each other, especially in the morning or while wanting attention, with the front feathers puffed up and out, giving the appearance of being in control and a bit fierce. It's the same expression they assumed while young in the nest, pretending they are bigger than they are.

Pigeons were first domesticated 5,000 years ago by Egyptians and used as message carriers. The Israelites, related in the Old Testament, often used pigeons as sacrificial animals in religious ceremonies.

Animal memory: You might be surprised

Most animal species have good homing instincts and will remember certain instances and happenings forever. If a young pup finds a way to crawl under or go through a break in a kennel fence, he'll soon find a way to get out again, no matter the repairs. Horses, cats, cattle, goats, pigs – the entire spectrum of animals and avian species – have the similar ability to remember home and how to escape again if confined. Rattlesnakes will home up to 20 miles from their den, returning to hibernate in a tangled mass during the cold winter months. In this situation, they are in a sort of tranquilized state of being and will not strike.

Monarch butterflies migrate from southern Canada and the north-central United States to central Mexico each fall. After a rest of five months spent clustered together to stay warm, they migrate north in spring and mate in the Southern states. The adults die and the newly metamorphic pupae, now as adult butterflies, continue north to their parents' ancestral homes, only to return again to Mexico in fall. The mystery, of course, is how these butterflies have the knowledge to return to the same place in Mexico, since only their genetic parents, not they themselves, were there the winter before. Animals are amazing creatures, as James Herriot implies in the title of his wonderful book *The Lord God Made Them All (All Creatures Great and Small).*

Skunked at age 6

One summer vacation day in 1934, the Menking bothers and I were playing near our farm when we saw a skunk go into a culvert about two feet in diameter. We decided to crawl in to try to catch it. We knew that skunks gave off a nasty odor, but had no idea just how nasty God had made these stinking kittens. The previously swampy farmland in Minnesota was drained years earlier, and large drainage culverts were plentiful.

There was not much drainage water in the summers of 1930s due to drought, and it was easy to find culverts free of water. Needless to say, we three boys got skunked. My mother was in a tirade and made us take off all of our clothes and get scrubbed down with soapy water containing baking soda and vinegar. We were dressed in my extra clothes, of which there were not many garments to go around.

When I was visiting Minnesota in 2004, Lloyd and Francis reminded me about the skunk incident. Obviously, humans can have great memories about certain incidences, especially when it comes to being skunked!

Injured again

In the winter of 1934, I was playing in the horse and cow barn with a large manure scoop shovel, pushing it forward while holding it against my lower right abdomen. Suddenly, I hit a small pile of frozen manure and the handle of the shovel abruptly pushed inward in my lower stomach area. The blow caused a severe tear of abdominal muscles. I was in pain and had an immediate swelling in the traumatized area. The county roads were blocked from a recent severe windy snowstorm, a frequent occurrence in Minnesota winters. That meant a diagnosis had to be made over the telephone, our only modern accessory. Dad talked with Dr. Rous, explaining in lay terms what had happened and describing the appearance of the swollen area.

Dr. Rous instructed Dad to have me lie on my back over the seat of a chair with my torso on the seat, and my head and legs dangling. If the swelling subsided, it would indicate a likely diagnosis of an abdominal rupture. That indeed proved to be the diagnosis; a few days later when the roads cleared I was able to see the doctor in Monte.

Following a snowstorm, a trip to Monte on a gravel road was not easy. It meant running the Model T Ford as fast as possible at snowdrifts, resulting in getting stuck again and again. There were no tire chains, which meant shoveling after every stall until the car was free, and then traveling at a maximum 10 mph until arriving at the state highway, where snow plows made the road passable to town. Minnesota Highway 7 was full of deep potholes, as road maintenance in those days was poor and the technology of building roads able to withstand severe winter weather had not been perfected.

Dr. Rous confirmed the diagnosis of abdominal rupture, with intestines coming through the muscle tears to the level of the skin. This type of tear was of major concern. Often with such ruptures, intestines become trapped and loss of blood supply results in necrosis (death of tissues), requiring intestinal anastomosis (surgical procedure to connect two sections of the intestines following removal of a diseased portion). Fortunately in my case, that did not happen. My treatment consisted of eight sessions with a sclerosing agent, which ordinarily is used to shrink varicose veins. The sclerosing solution was injected at weekly intervals into the area of the rupture with a needle that looked like a large dagger. A rubber-balled truss was used to hold the intestines out of the ruptured area until healing, induced by the injections, took place. Although I clearly remember those injections as painful, I did not shed a tear.

The rupture healed, and I never had evidence of a recurring tear. Abdominal surgery was not attempted because my parents simply did not have money for such an operation in the deep Depression of 1934. In 2006, I had an abdominal MRI, which showed evidence of calcified scar tissue in the area of the hernia that Dr. Rous had treated 74 years earlier. I suspect that such a treatment in the modern medical era would be considered malpractice.

Modern veterinary and human health-care availability and delivery have dramatically changed since the 1930s–1950s era. The federal government began this process in the 1960s with development of Medicare. This led at the same time to development of private health care insurance coverage as physician fees and costs associated with medical technology and hospital care were rising dramatically. By the turn of the new millennium, the cost of health care had become a matter of national concern. There is no way to re-employ the one-to-one doctor-patient relationships common during my childhood, when medical costs were often paid by the barter system with farm produce. There were no third-party insurance companies or federal government safety nets.

Veterinary medicine tended to be more affordable until the 1990s, when costs began to skyrocket. In the new millennium, veterinary health costs have proportionally followed the huge increases in human medical health delivery. It is now increasingly difficult to provide veterinary medical care for the pets of middle-class citizens, but animal health insurance helps by encouraging better contact with veterinarians. Clinical trials and other clinical research have become increasingly difficult to conduct in comparison to development of veterinary cancer medicine in the 1970s.

Abuzz about honeybees

During an outing with the Menking brothers in the summer of 1935, we went three miles from their farm to pick crab apples. I have cherished these delicious little red fruits my whole life. We found beehives in the crab apple orchard, and inquisitiveness led to desire for honey.

In order to get to the honey, I tipped over a hive. My-oh-my, did the bees swarm at us as we ran away, frightened, yelling at the top of our lungs and getting stung many times. Luckily, none of us

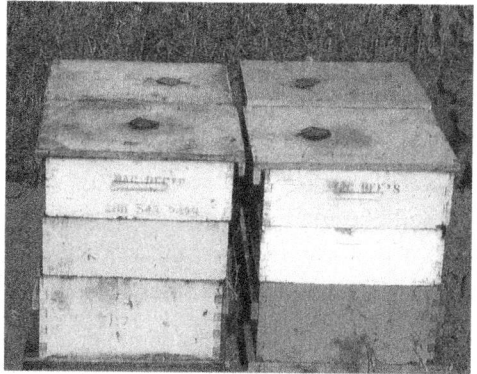

Beehive with supers (boxes to hold bee combs with wax and honey) in 2016, similar to a hive Gordon tipped over in 1935 (Photo by Christine Ortego).

were allergic to bee stings, but our heads and arms were swollen way beyond normal. A photograph would have made a good record of the event.

Tina Menking was very upset with us when we returned to their farm. Francis brought the memory to the surface when I visited Minnesota in 2003.

To tell the truth, I did not need to be reminded of the incident or my juvenile lack of judgment.

In the 1980s, I became an apiarist and began a few beehives. I learned that after a few months, bees recognized me and I could be around their hives and not be attacked by guard bees. This is interesting, because bees do not live very long. By the time I was accepted near the hives, the original bees would have been dead. What interesting facts one learns when becoming aware of the biological plans of plants, insects, and higher forms of life!

Bees are special insects, mentioned in the Bible, and have been of use to humans for thousands of years. When the Israelites left Egypt and were in the wilderness for 40 years, they finally found the land of "milk and honey" in Judea and elsewhere in Israel. Honey is a special food that in storage does not spoil, and acts like an antibiotic. It is wound-healing and of considerable value to health when consumed as a regular part of diet. My grandfather Henry Theilen kept bees, and he and grandma always had honey on their dining table. Pa started his apiary by collecting a hive that had taken up residence between the walls in their attic. He did this when the hive was swarming. With the hatch of a new queen, the bees that were attracted to her swarmed and left the hive with her.

Swarming bees will not sting, and thousands can be on a person without harm. Thus, Pa could place the new colony in a man-made hive, where they quickly took up residence. Bees naturally select or are placed in an enclosure that is of a certain volume to meet their needs. Worker bees set up new hives in suitably proportioned spaces such as hollowed-out trees, logs, or human-constructed areas such as the space between the walls in my grandfather's attic.

The queen has drones that work for her, collecting pollen to become honey. Guard bees protect the hive. Worker bees, always female, will go as far as 10 miles from the hive and do not have the ability to sting. If a hive is moved just a few feet while the worker bees are out, they are unable to find it when they return. But if one moves the hive more than 10 miles away and then releases the worker bees, they are able to find the hive just fine. This is another very interesting example of animals' truly amazing homing instinct.

Bees are necessary for pollination of certain agricultural crops, including almond trees, which without their help will not bear fruit. Interestingly enough, bees that are used to pollinate almond orchards are imported to California from Minnesota each year in early January or February, when the trees bloom. As spring progresses, they are returned to Minnesota for use with other crops. For travel, the entrance to the hives is blocked until the journey is complete. Bees help farmers around the world produce billions of dollars worth of produce each year. An immune deficiency syndrome is affecting bee populations worldwide. In some areas of China bees have disappeared, and humans now must perform pollination.

Thieves in the neighborhood

One evening in 1936 after being away and coming home after dark, we found the family dog, Rex, a German shepherd, tied up and most of Mom's chickens missing. Some neighbors living close to our farm, apparently were the thieves; shortly after we arrived, we heard their car leaving over gravel a mile away. After that, Rex always growled at them when they were in the vicinity of our farm. It is amazing how dogs remember and equate related occurrences with uncanny accuracy.

We also had a smaller, terrier-type dog, Tricksy. One day Tricksy and Rex were gone all day. Late that night, Rex came home but Tricksy did not. Rex beckoned dad to follow him. In a nearby farm field, they came to a badger hole. We believe that is where the little dog met her demise. Rex was despondent after that for some time. He had sired a litter of pups with Tricksy. We kept a male puppy, King. He looked mostly shepherd. Unfortunately, he developed distemper at an early age, suffered encephalitic seizures, and never was healthy. He recovered from the seizures but was always listless with diminished value as a guard dog.

Move to the Schield farm

We had moved from the Thompson farm near Maynard to the Schield farm three miles north of Montevideo on March 1, 1937, after a snowstorm that left drifts as high as telephone poles, with no fence lines to be seen. I do not remember much about my sister Blythe's childhood before age 3, when she returned with grandparents that spring of 1937 from a visit with relatives. She had a deep chest cough, a high fever and was in a depressed mood. She said to my parents "I don't feel well, Mommy and Daddy."

They took Blythe to see Dr. Rous the same day, and she was diagnosed with pneumonia involving both lungs. She was hospitalized immediately in the Monte hospital for a week before her fever of 106 degrees Fahrenheit broke. The state highway was made passable by plows that pushed the snow into walls 12 feet high on either side of the road.

What a way to begin life as sharecroppers on a new farm! The snow from that storm lasted up to the time Blythe was in the hospital with pneumonia. Very cold and rainy weather persisted through April. The beginning of our life on the Schield farm was as unusually bad economically as climatically.

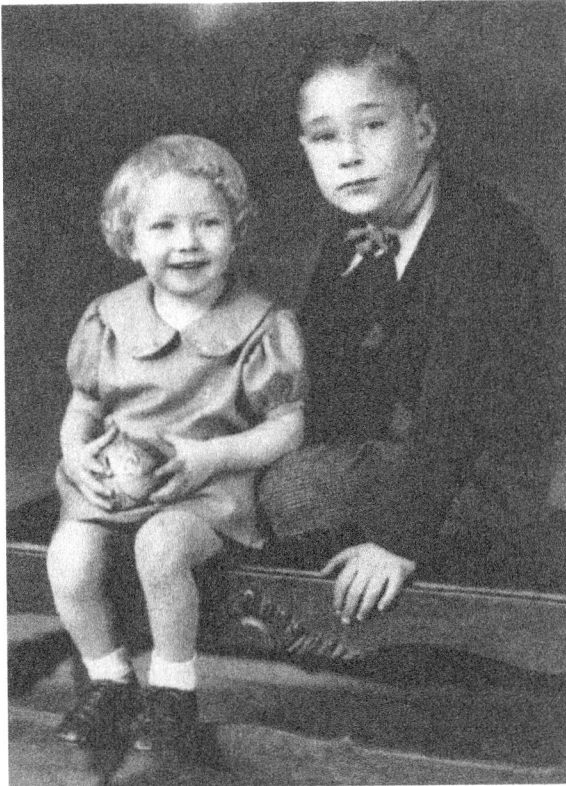

Blythe, age 3, and me, age 8.

CHAPTER 5

Bitter Cold

"Attitude is a little thing that makes a big difference."
– Winston Churchill

Snowstorm, 1938

One very cold February morning in 1938, after a severe snowstorm, Mom said to Dad, "Should we let Gordon go to school today?" Dad replied, "He's a tough boy. No problem, he can make it."

We were living on the Schield farm, just south of the Behren farm, about three miles north of Monte. I was never pampered, given leeway in life experiences. On that cold February morning, the world was extremely still. There was no breeze, and the snow level was higher than field fences. All was awesomely quiet. It seemed like the Earth had stood still following the blizzard of the night before.

The sun shone brightly, producing tiny reflections of color spectrum glittering from trillions of snowflakes. The effect was like myriad tiny rainbows strewn across an infinite white landscape. The harsh environment had been transformed, at least for a while, into a winter wonderland.

On this clear day, walking was challenging. With every step, I heard the crunch of my overshoes on fresh snow. There were no other sounds to be

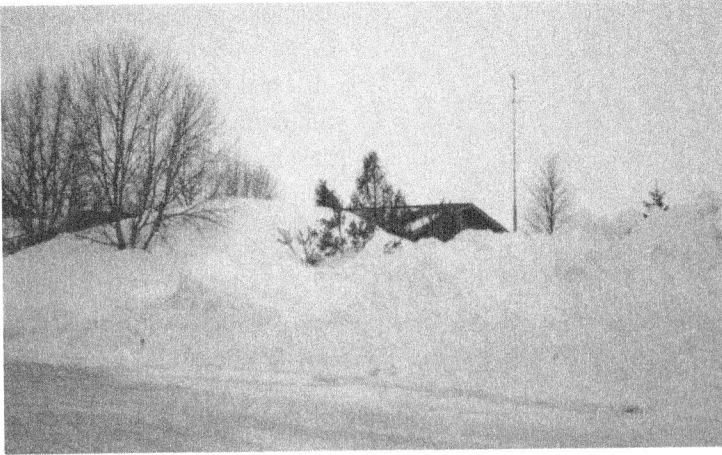

Minnesota scene after a severe snowstorm (Compliments of Mrs. Nola Sulflow).

heard. Luckily, the snow was crusted enough so that my feet sank only an inch or two below the surface. I remembered the step-after-step, crunch-after-crunch sensation of walking to school that day.

I was 10, and the temperature was 30 degrees below zero. What a wonderful experience it was to arrive at school and be embraced by the warmth of a coal-burning stove. I deposited my overshoes, mittens, scarf, snow mask, and heavy coat in the coatroom. Long underwear, a wool shirt and farmer-type coveralls were sufficient to maintain body heat at my assigned desk. The potbelly stove, aglow with warmth, was in the front of the room near the teacher's desk.

The teacher, a young, single woman, remarked, "Gordon, you had quite a walk this morning, didn't you? Several of your student friends did not make it to school today." The school had a student body of 12, with only eight in attendance that day. The reduced number of students gave me a feeling of "making it" while others could not navigate the deep snow.

Most kids in those days had chilblains, a tissue injury of the feet caused by prolonged exposure to cold and humidity. Chilblains created soreness, especially around the heel area, leading to reddened inflammation that did not easily heal and go away because of continued exposure to the elements and recurring freezing of the skin. Other areas of the body where wet clothing froze also developed problems. Feet were frequently wet due to damaged overshoes and shoes that did not shed water. Chilblains were especially painful when

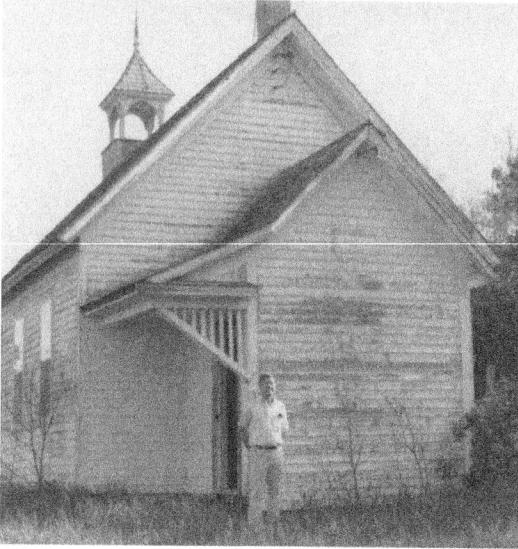

That's me in 1997 at the Chippewa County, Rosewood Township District 25 one-room school I attended 1936–1939.

warming feet quickly next to the stove. Many students also had frostbite of the ears, fingertips, and cheeks. Minnesota was very cold from November through most of March.

During morning and afternoon recesses, which were just 10 minutes long, kids would have snowball fights to take off some of the pent-up energy that resulted from being in a one-room building from 9 a.m. to 4 p.m. Occasionally, a frozen snowball would hit a student foe in the head, causing injury. Snow forts would be built, and one team would attack the other, with all boys and girls participating in the snowball battles.

Toilets were outhouses, one for the boys and one for the girls. If a student needed to go to the toilet, a raised hand with one finger up meant request to urinate, and two, request to defecate. I don't clearly recall why indication for one or the other was required, but it must have had to do with discipline. Going to the toilet in subfreezing cold was enormously unpleasant. The toilets were not heated, and were as cold on the inside as on the outside. Toilet paper was not available; we used pages from mail-order catalogs that parents donated. Catalog paper was not absorbent, and its slick edges could cause skin lacerations. In the wintertime, heavily insulated coveralls and long underwear had to be lowered in order to sit on the cold seats. Needless to say, the teacher did not check on what a student was doing, because it was too cold to stay outside more than a minute or two. Loitering did not occur in the wintertime.

The terror of tornadoes

While winters in Minnesota were very cold, summers could be hot and humid. Tornadoes occasionally occurred. The heart of the tornado belt was

32

farther south, but twisters did touch down in our area and wreak havoc. One I remember with clarity occurred on Memorial Day 1938, several miles east of where we lived. At our farm, we experienced an electrical storm with repeated lightning strikes accompanied by horrendous thunderclaps, churning winds and hailstones the size of marbles and larger. My uncle Harold Sufflow was at the time feeding milk from a pail to a calf with its head in a metal stanchion. Lightning struck the barn, which was grounded, but electricity ran along the metal manure-bucket carrier, jumped about six feet from there to the metal stanchion and killed the calf instantly. My uncle, holding the metal bucket from which the calf had been drinking seconds before, was unharmed.

The tornado hit nearby locales harder, destroying buildings, uprooting trees, and propelling blades of grass with enough force to puncture car tires. The date of this storm, May 31, sticks in my mind because we had just returned from visiting relatives' graves in Granite Falls, Minnesota. Every year on Memorial Day, gravesites were beautified and flowers were planted in fond memory of relatives and friends. I'd had a wonderful 10th birthday celebration the day before, and was terror-struck by the fury of the storm. While we were not in the direct path of the tornado, just being in proximity was a fearful experience.

Changing times, 1936–1939

Discipline meted out at school varied, but a slap on the rear or the back of the hand from a foot-long ruler was a common punishment for the younger students in grades one through four. Students from fifth through eighth grades were verbally disciplined or grounded from recesses and other types of pleasure. Today's students have breaks from school for entire days or weeks, and occasional school-sponsored field trips for educational purposes. There were no days off or field trips from the one-room school.

One spring day in May 1938, not long before summer recess, I was swinging on the school flagpole and bent it into a "C" shape. The schoolmarm was irate and indicated that, to stay in school, I had to obtain permission from all three school-board members. These men were all farmers in the area. I rode a bicycle for several miles to obtain signatures in order to avoid expulsion. I never told my parents about that, and it was never discussed. As far as I knew, my parents never found out about the gravity of the situation. I felt humiliated, much like a beaten dog, and wanted to hide from this awful event. I suspect the teacher and trustees all told my parents, but it always remained a secret. It was obvious the reason for secrecy was to avoid additional wrath from home, and perhaps I pulled off the coup and my parents never learned of my disgrace.

Animal breeding: My sex education

One of my early farming experiences involved bringing a purebred Belgian stallion to the Schield farm to breed one of Dad's mares, Dolly, a crossbreed with some Western bronco blood. The stallion, chestnut with a light-colored mane, showed his masculinity by snorting, rearing, and acting up. He knew there was a mare in season to breed.

Many farm youngsters were not allowed to witness animal mating. It was a subject never discussed. Stallions were brought by their owners to breed a mare. Dad had mixed breeds of horses that were crosses of draft breeds with wild mustangs from the Dakotas, Wyoming, and Montana. These horses were crossed with purebred draft horses, usually Belgian, Percheron, shire, or Clydesdale. The owner brought the stallion in a specially built rig that resembled a horse trailer placed on top of a truck bed. The truck was a late 1920s or early 1930s model, and the passenger stallion was easily visible to passersby. The stallion was very aggressive and eager to mate the mare in season. Often, when two horses are put together to breed, the mare is unwilling and human assistance is needed. As a veterinarian years later, I often was in charge of breeding horses. But when I first witnessed the endeavor, I was a mere boy just 7 years old.

Dad did not talk to me about birds and bees when I reached puberty. What I knew about sex I learned in a practical way by witnessing the mating of horses, cattle, pigs, sheep and poultry, all part of life on a farm, the way of perpetuating species. Later, perpetuation was commonly accomplished by artificial insemination of cooled or frozen semen given to females in receptive estrus cycle. The development of artificial insemination replaced male animals with technically trained humans on many farms. The domesticated turkey has been so genetically altered that the male (tom) can no longer physically mate with the female. To perpetuate, all females must be fertilized by artificial insemination. Modern technology has altered many ways of life.

CHAPTER 6

All About a Mule and Horses

"Never look backwards or you'll fall down the stairs."
– Rudyard Kipling

Wanting a pony

When I was a boy I longed for a riding horse, but never had the gift of having one. As a youngster, I often dreamed of getting a Shetland pony, but when I awakened, none was there. My family relocated to the Schield farm when I was in the third grade. It was here, at age 9, that I started to become a responsible person, helping on the farm in many ways. These were hard times financially, and my parents struggled to stay solvent in farming and to keep food on the table. It was a drought year. Home vegetable gardens dried up, field crops failed, and prices fell to record lows.

This meant little time for entertainment and only time for work, which was accomplished with horse-drawn implements and human hand labor. I was allowed to ride Dad's draft horses on Sundays and times of the year when they were not overly worked. I had a few minor accidents while riding bareback, as the horse invariably would gallop when turning for home, and I invariably would fall off. Later in life, I had several horse accidents. One in 1985 nearly led to my demise.

A foreshadowing incident

I had just returned from a speaking engagement in Germany and Switzerland, after giving a seminar in Berne on discovery of the feline sarcoma virus (Snyder-Theilen feline sarcoma virus, the first domesticated mammalian sarcoma virus to be discovered), and immunological research conducted with the virus. (The process of discovering the first feline sarcoma virus will be discussed in detail in my book *One Medicine War on Cancer*).

Before returning to Frankfurt the next day by train for connection to San Francisco, I was invited to swim in the Aare River. It swiftly flows from the snow-covered Alps traversing Berne. This was the first time I had ever swum in a fast-moving current. The entry point was a set of steps in a city park. Upon entering the water, the idea was to swim swiftly downstream with the fast current, then maneuvering by side-paddling to exit steps on the shore. A path led back to the entry point upstream.

Close call on the Lochsa

That learning experience saved my life a month later in Idaho. I had planned an elk-hunting trip with a former student of mine, Clarence Binninger, DVM, M.S. We rendezvoused at his home in Lewiston, Idaho, to ready for a horse pack trip into the Bitterroot Mountains, at a place near Missoula, Montana. We drove his truck 100 miles, carrying four horses and gear needed for a week, and unloaded near the Lochsa River.

Two horses were used for packing and two for riding. Crossing the river at 4,000 feet elevation was necessary to access the mountain trail leading to the hunting spike camp established at 7,000 feet. Clarence crossed first, leading a pack horse and riding a strong saddle horse. I followed, leading a young pack horse and riding a reliable older gelding named Chico, a relatively small horse measuring 14 hands. While following Clarence from sandbar to sandbar, Chico was swept off his feet by the swift current. Together, in no time, we were swept into rapids in the upper reaches of the Lochsa. It took experience to survive swimming in swift rapids, especially wearing heavy boots and wool clothing needed at high elevation during the September elk-hunting season.

As we were swept down the river 200 yards, we were caught in a clear, swift current that pushed us toward the opposite shore. I grabbed a large boulder and immediately slipped off while hollering "Oh shiiittt!" Almost instantly, I grabbed onto another boulder and was able, with brute strength, to hold on with legs forced into a position parallel to the swift water exerting unbelievable pull downstream. Just a few yards beyond was another set of rapids with steeper falls and obvious threatening consequences. Experience I had gained swimming in the Aare River a month earlier led to my miraculous survival, and Chico was spared, as well. My guardian angel had grabbed me and aided me in garnering enough energy and strength to pull myself to safety and wave to Clarence, who was upstream about a third of a mile.

I was safe and sound, but completely soaked. Chico, standing behind a boulder in calm eddy of water, had to be unsaddled and swum upstream alongside the high cliffs that prevented walking on the shore. Clarence said later he was thinking, as he watched me flounder about, what he should say to Carolyn. At the time, he surely thought I would not survive.

The experience of being swept through rushing water rapids, sucked under again and again, is unforgettable. The Lord had a plan for me to continue to have my heart beat an additional 86,400 times a day for many more years, which amounts to several billion beats and counting since my conception in 1928. It is an amazing how God provides a means to survive horrific accidents.

Survival instinct is pronounced in all animals no matter what obstacles are presented. What marvelous order and synchrony given by the Master Architect who knitted our bodies together with laminins. The chemical makeup of this protein network, when pictorially depicted, is in the design of a cross. I was saved to live and continue into eternity by the Cross.

Another tumble

I've experienced many other horse accidents, but none as horrific as being swept downstream on the Lochsa. However, quadriceps and groin pulls I experienced in a fall later in life never fully cured. That most recent accident occurred a day before I underwent total knee replacement surgery on May 5, 2007. I was in the saddle on Chance, my Missouri fox-trotter gelding, at Red Rock Field Trial Grounds, a 20-degree sloping mountainous field-trial area north of Reno, Nevada.

Chance froze, and when I gently gave him a spur, he reared. I immediately tried to rein him to the side to prevent him from rearing high. Unfortunately, I reined him to the down side of the mountain, and that tipped him over. As he was falling, I cast off the saddle. Side-by-side we rolled near each other for 15 yards before coming to a stop. Chance got up and stood. I had tremendous pain in my right quadriceps and had a severe groin pull with pain that made mounting up for two-mile ride to camp difficult.

I took two Tylenol tablets upon return to camp. Many friends wondered if they should call 911. Of course, I refused. I still was having difficulty walking the next day, though, when my journalist friend Janet Fullwood brought me home. I had to be at the Sutter Hospital the day after that for total replacement of my left knee. A family friend, Sharon Jahn, drove me to the hospital for my 5 a.m. appointment. I had difficulty walking on my left leg because of knee arthritis and on the right due to muscle and ligament damage two days prior to total knee replacement. That was a painful morning before my 7 a.m. surgery.

The surgeon, Dr. David Coward, asked if I felt in condition to have a knee replacement, and I answered "yes." Dr. Coward did not know of the horse accident and groin injury until several weeks later, when I was to begin rehab. I needed physical therapy of the right leg, but never received it. Ever since, the leg has been stiff and sore each morning.

Saying goodbye to Derby

My favorite mount for 15 years was not a horse, but rather was Derby, my loyal Molly mule. In June 2006, at age 78, I was forced to have my wonderful and close riding companion euthanized due to severe arthritis. I experienced an emotional event that equated to the loss of a dear human friend. I held Derby's lead as a concentrated barbiturate was intravenously administered by a veterinary colleague. She quickly fell and crumpled to the ground in front of the "Boy

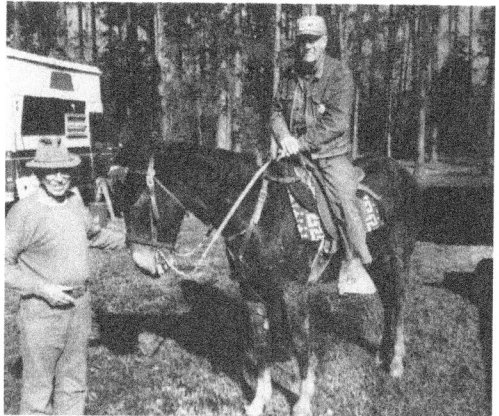

Derby, a friend, and me in 1994 at the Brittany All Age Nationals at Blue Mountain Hunting Preserve in Booneville, Arkansas.

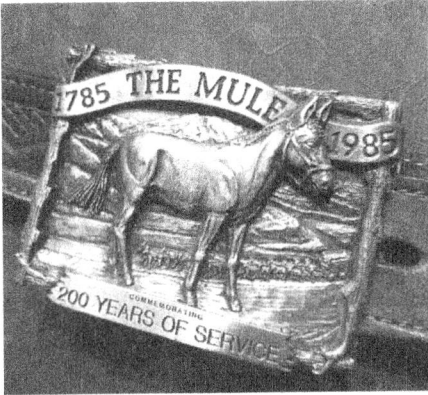

Belt buckle commemorating 200 years of (mule) service to the United States.

With the Wounded Thumb." Tears were shed. Derby and I were firmly bonded, and she left a void that never again was filled. Derby was the only gaited mule I would ever own and experience pleasure in riding. Age was a factor and I couldn't justify the purchase of another mule or additional horses.

Interestingly, the king of Spain gave two male jackasses to our first president, George Washington. He bred the jacks to some of his finest mares in 1785. This started the breeding of mules in the newly formed nation. Mules helped build our nation's infrastructure. They were hardier than horses, and could work in desert and semi-desert areas of the country where horses couldn't, as well as help break sod in development of our agricultural enterprises elsewhere.

Learning to swim

I learned to swim after the move to the Schield farm in 1936. The local swimming hole was a recreational area at the confluence of the Minnesota and Chippewa rivers in Montevideo's Smith Park. There was a lifeguard and an anchored raft that kids could swim to and have fun. I learned to dive from a tree limb on the opposite shore into the river.

I rode a bicycle three miles from the farm to go swimming. The bike was a gift from Aunt Florence, my mother's oldest sister. She was single and doted over me as if I were her son. On hot summer days, when temperatures sometimes topped 100 degrees, I would stop at the Schallenbergers' farm, about halfway to the swimming hole, for a cool drink of water. On the return trip, I'd stop again at the shady farmhouse with its well-insulated water-tank house. Often, Mrs. Schallenberger would have cold lemonade available for me. The Schallenbergers were childless and really took to me, a youngster of 9. This was almost like heaven.

Aunt Florence and Mrs. Schallenberger were not my only sources of spoiling. My Schaller grandparents spoiled me the most. I was Henry and Millie Schaller's first grandchild, and Grandpa Schaller saw no fault with me. My grandmother was a stern disciplinarian, but my grandfather, affectionately known as Hank, was never strict. Hank was a hardworking farmer who always made time for me as a youngster. Grandma Schaller was a wonderful, hardworking housewife and able assistant in farming, milking cows, and doing all the needed vegetable-garden work in summer. She always kept a neat home; one of a special kind, she never complained, and was always positive in support of her family. I had special relationship with her and loved her very much, as she taught me patience, dedication and responsibility.

I never forgot our last meeting. She was 84 and in an assisted living facility, Luther Haven, in Monte. It was the summer of 1965, and when saying goodbye, I knew it was for the last time. She was always jovial and said, "Gordon, you know what I would like most at this time?" "What, Grandma?" "To have a family picnic." Family picnics happened once or twice a year, with all family members getting together to have fun and share experiences. The best time for a picnic was on May 31, Memorial Day, when the dead were remembered and flowers were placed on gravesites.

Tears came down my cheeks as I walked away from our meeting, knowing this was the last time I would ever see my beloved grandmother. Our son Kyle, then 10 years old, long remembered those tears streaming down the face of his father who never shed tears. Grandma Millie was a special woman who helped shape my life. I recall with amazing clarity the many experiences of staying overnight with Grandma and Grandpa Schaller in the noticeably cold upstairs bedroom. "Gordon, would you like to sleep under the horse blanket tonight?" Grandma would ask.

Grandma gave that blanket to me shortly before she died. I have it as a covering now on the living room couch. The blanket was made from the hide of one of their draft horses, a bay-colored animal of the shire breed. The hide was tanned and had a wool felt backing attached, with the Schaller name and the name of the maker sewn on. It was made way back in the late 1890s and used on a regular basis up until the horse-drawn buggy and sleigh was replaced by automobiles in the late 1920s. My mother related that she, along with her siblings, used the blanket to cover their legs in winter when the family went to church on Sunday mornings. The blanket now serves mostly as a covering for the couch and conversation piece of historical interest. Our pet cat, Bobbie, a tabby Manx female with white paws, sleeps on it. On occasion, granddaughters cover themselves with it, too. It is more than 100 years old and still looks like the blanket I slept under as a very young boy.

Family history

My Schaller grandparents were first-generation German Americans who spoke broken English and were devout Christians. They lived according to Christian beliefs the best they could. My grandmother was an angel the Lord placed on Earth. Carolyn, my wife, was gifted by an angel and the best woman I ever knew, even better than grandmas Millie Schaller, Meta Theilen, and my mother. I consider myself fortunate for outstanding women in my life.

My mother was frequently depressed and I was often uncomfortable with her in company; she acted strangely at times. These behaviors were most acute during my early childhood. She became less afflicted with strange behavior as I grew older. She was charming with high school friends, and most of the time

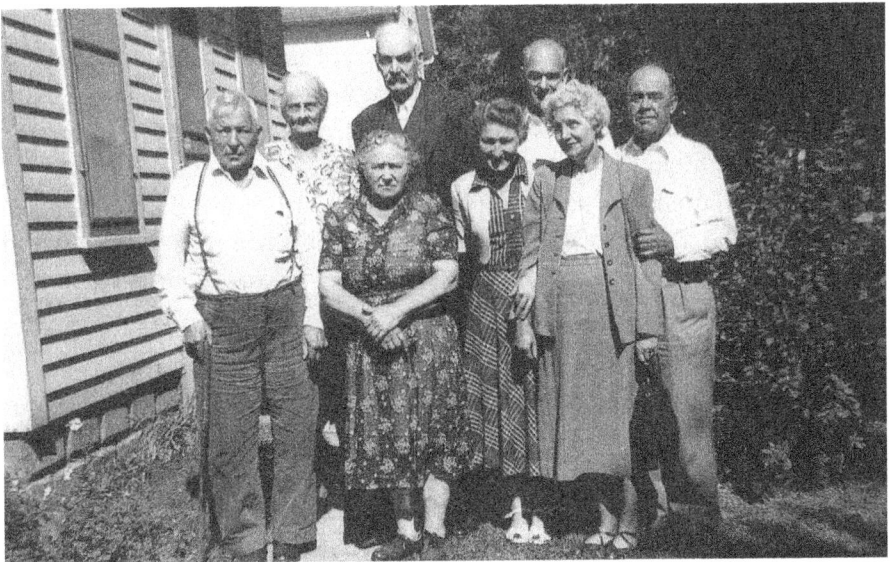

This 1949 family snapshot shows, in the back row, left to right, Grandma and Grandpa Theilen, Dad (Lou Theilen), and Uncle Frank Scholer In the front row, left to right, are Grandpa and Grandma Schaller, Mom, Ema Theilen, and Aunt Emma Scholer.

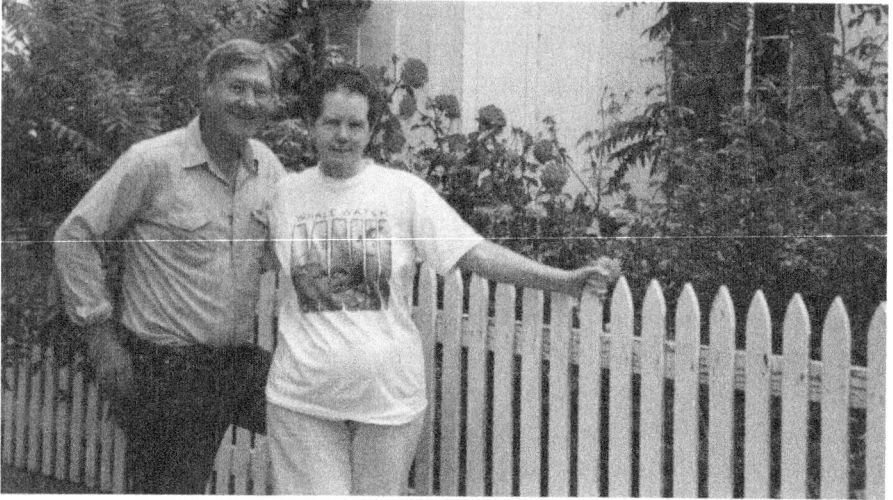

Carolyn and me in 1994 alongside the rose garden at our then-newly purchased retirement home near Dixon, California.

with others. Her condition became more noticeable from the time I returned from the Army until my dad died in 1965. She then took hold of her normal self again and was relatively free of severe depression attacks.

Despite health problems, Mom was a dedicated mother and wife and worked efficiently as a housewife, keeping our home in order. Early in marriage she labored at farm work as most women were needed as a farmhand. Dad was not as energetic as Mom and consequently was not a tirelessly dedicated farmer. He probably did not like the farming environment because he was afflicted with asthma and hay fever, and as a teenager probably had polio. He developed a lasting limp that followed a bout of illness when he was 12 years old.

Dust storms, crop failures, and being forced to sell good-quality milk cows for $15 each were discouraging circumstances for a man trying to raise a family and keep a business. There was little hope of solvency, because a sharecropper was in bondage to farm ownership. The reality of sharecrop farming during the Depression years initiated motivation to sell belongings and move West. It was a lure that had beckoned Dad ever since he'd spent two years, from 1920 to 1922, working in the lumber industry near Port Angeles, Washington. He talked glowingly about the West Coast. Thus, after a farming partnership with his uncle Ben Theilen failed in the spring of 1939, it was easy for him to call farming quits.

We lived through June with the Schaller grandparents. Mom came down with a kidney illness and could not travel until early August. I traveled by train from Maynard to Le Mars, Iowa, and stayed with Aunt and Uncle Scholer. My dad's sister had married Frank Scholer, and my Mother's maiden name was Schaller. Le Mars was Dad's hometown, and many relative lived in and around Le Mars and the farming area in Grant Township, near Sioux City. I had a wonderful time with my cousins Darrel and Bud Scholer. We spent a lot of time each day swimming at White Way swimming hole, an old sand pit. I fondly remember uncle Frank Scholer, who was Plymouth County sheriff, frequently taking us out to dinner at the Pantry. My favorite dish was a pork-roast sandwich with massive amounts of white gravy.

The Scholer family resided in the living quarters of the county jail. A door led from the kitchen to the cellblock. Emma, my aunt, prepared meals for the prisoners, and I passed the food on a tray through a portal in the jail door. I frequently talked with the prisoners. Few were hard-core criminals. Most were alcoholics or accused of running booze from states that permitted possession of alcoholic beverages. Iowa did not. It was referred to as a blue-law state. Many Iowans did not obey the repeal of Prohibition in 1932. Hence, one cell in the jail was devoted to storing alcoholic beverages taken from persons who had possessed them illegally.

When the Scholers visited us in Minnesota, Uncle Frank would bring a fifth or two to Dad. The Scholers did not drink alcoholic beverages, and Dad and Mom did so infrequently, usually when going once or twice a year to barn dances. Kids were brought along and would dance on the sidelines while the adults square-danced, waltzed, or did other Northern European-type dances.

Young boy needed for farm labor

In the years from 1936 to 1939, I became a needed farmhand and participated in feeding stock, cleaning the barn and helping in castrating piglets. I also fixed fences to prevent milk cows from escaping into nearby cornfields where they would gorge themselves and develop bloat that led to death. My mother and I would chase the cows back into a pasture that was in poor grazing grass condition because of low rainfall and lack of reseeding. In the mid 1930s, Minnesota suffered from severe drought, as the Great Plains states did. Nevertheless, poor crops were harvested. It was exciting for me to experience the threshing of oats, wheat, barley, and flax, all with their different fragrances. Wheat and flax were highly aromatic, while oats and barley had more subdued scents.

Six or so farmers formed into a threshing crew, and with a team of horses and a wagon would help each other bring shocked (harvested) grain to the thresher for separation of grain and straw. The straw was blown from the thresher onto a stack 10 to 12 feet high and was used for animal winter bedding. Grain was elevated to the granary, or taken to town and stored in huge silos along the railroad tracks for immediate sale.

On one trip to Monte, riding with a farmer taking grain to the granary, the old Model A Ford truck could hardly make a slight grade on the state highway and chugged forward at 5 mph or so. Upon reaching town and while waiting to unload the grain, I recall farmers talking about the serious matter of Nazi Germany invading Czechoslovakia, and what seemed like imminent war. A 15-year-old, low-IQ lad added to the conversation. "I don't care if the United States goes to war, but sure hope Minnesot (slang for Minnesota) stays out," he said, revealing a glimpse of the rural worldview.

Hitler's plans were not known at that time, and we all thought the threat of war would just go away. However, it did not, as we found out on December 7, 1941, when the Japanese bombed Pearl Harbor. President Roosevelt immediately declared war on the Japanese Empire. Soon afterward, Germany and Italy, both allies of Japan, declared war on the United States, enveloping the world in war.

Threshing crews

One day during dinner for the threshing crew, an incident occurred. Mrs. Nelson brought food to the table for the crew and said, "Men, I have been beaning you to death for the last few days, and now will pea you to death." That innocent comment is well remembered, as it raised a wave of laughter from the threshing crew.

My Great Uncle John Theilen, Dad's uncle and youngest brother of my grandfather Henry Theilen, was a thresher who lived in Grant Township, Iowa. He hired out his services to farmers throughout the Midwest region, starting the season in Texas in early summer, moving gradually north with his steam-

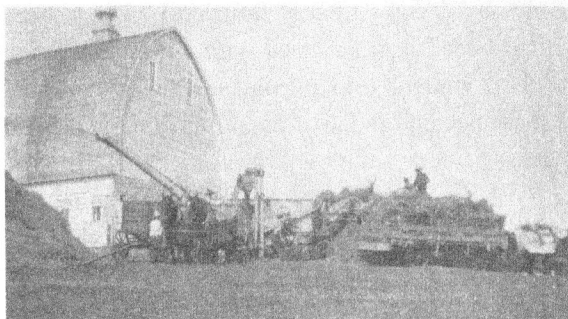

Distant shot of thresher, with team left attached to wagon collecting grain. Right team was hitched to wagon with man tossing bundles of grain onto a conveyer belt to send bundles to the thresher to separate grain and straw blown to stack, left.

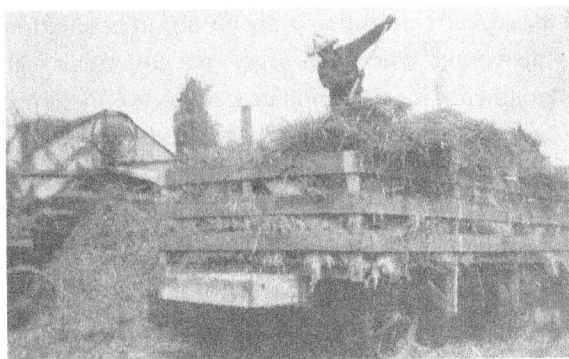

Close-up of bundles thrown on converyer belt to thresher (Compliments of Odell Schaller, Maynard, MN).

driven tractor and threshing machine, reaching Minnesota and Iowa in late August and continuing on to Manitoba, Canada, in September. He would then go back to western Iowa and work on the machinery, getting ready for the next year's threshing in Texas.

Corn was a major crop that had to be hand-picked (shucked) and thrown into a side-boarded wagon pulled by a team of horses. The horses were trained to stop thousands of times a day, and to move forward by "get up" and "wow." Picked corn was brought to the granary, shelled, and elevated to the storage area.

A sled accident

A 10-foot-high straw stack made from threshing became a place of play in the winter. It would be covered with snow and served as a windbreak. Cattle would eat vertically up to the highest point they could reach, turning their side of the stack into a vertical wall. One day, I was sledding down the sloping side of the stack and decided it would be real neat to climb to the top, zoom over the vertical drop of about eight feet and continue sledding at the bottom. Instead, I slammed violently to the ground at the bottom of the stack. My nose at the bridge was cut through the nasal turbinates, with two holes opening to the edge of the ethmoid plate separating the nasal passages from the brain.

As I got up, Dad heard me say, "Wow, almost broke my neck." Then the cold air hit my brain as if I'd been hit in the head with a sledgehammer. I immediately was in severe pain, with blood squirting out the wound and covering my face. The white snow became red as if an animal's main carotid artery had been cut in slaughter.

Dad rushed with me to the house and said to Mom, "Ema [Mom spelled her first name with one "m"] we have to immediately take Gordon to Dr. Rous. He has severely injured himself, and I can see his brain." Of course, it was the ethmoid plate, but for one uninformed about human anatomy, it was not too far off. Only a few millimeters of bony tissue separated what he saw from the brain proper. I have never forgotten the severe headache that resulted from the subzero cold air hitting the ethmoid directly, then through the nasal turbinate passageway to trachea and lungs.

Dr. Rous cleaned the wound, applied antiseptic – probably an iodine solution – and taped a bandage across the wound. It healed nicely, but a noticeable scar at the bridge of the nose has remained. This was another example of my living on the fringe and doing the unexpected. Even though sliding 90 degrees off a snow-covered straw stack and over an eight-foot precipice was dumb and lacked good judgment, it took courage as I all the while imagined I would be propelled onward – were it not for the force of gravity.

CHAPTER 7

More Tissue Scars

"I've just learned about his illness. Let's hope it's nothing trivial."

– Irvin S. Cobb

Accidental and surgical

The nasal scar left by the straw stack accident was my third-largest, following the scar I carried from almost losing my right thumb and the deep gash in my left kneecap incurred while I was chasing a floating-away lunch bucket. More injuries were to come.

As a high-school football player, I sustained another scar from being cleated in the left eyebrow. While playing sandlot baseball in Richmond, California, in 1943, a hard pitch hit me in the left ear, imprinting the seam of the ball on my face and knocking out an upper left incisor, leaving the nerve exposed. I underwent a root canal, and although I really needed a false tooth, that nerveless root remained intact until I was in my 60s. Finally at that time Dr. Jim Davis, an outstanding dentist in Davis, California, extracted the tooth and constructed a bridge that lasted 25 years. In 2011, it was replaced with another bridge supported by two titanium tooth implants.

Another small scar is a reminder of an injury I sustained in the early 1960s while doing veterinary work on the Ackermann dairy near Orland, California. I was suturing a cow's teat when she kicked back, forcing my right arm against a rear squeeze shoot support and sending pain shooting instantly to my shoulder. The arm then went numb. This injury proved to be a muscle tear in a "U" shape of about 10 centimeters above the wrist without a skin tear. Interestingly, a scar formed and has remained since.

Knee replacement

The only surgical scar I sustained up to 83 years of age was a 20-centimeter mark resulting from total left knee replacement that Dr. David Coward performed at Sutter General Hospital in Sacramento on May 14, 2007. I had experienced soreness in the knee for several years before that. He had helped the large-animal clinic at the UC Davis veterinary school initiate arthroscopic joint examinations in horses, and he treated several colleagues of mine for knee problems. His brother was a former student who became an equine practitioner. On my first visit to Dr. Coward, he indicated he could relieve the pain by intra-articular cortisone injections. I was opposed to injection of corticosteroid because it led to severe arthritis in horses. He immediately replied, "You are not a horse."

He gave injections once every four to six months, and let the injection results dictate time for surgery. Within 15 minutes of joint-fluid removal and injection, I could walk on the leg and apply body weight to the joint without pain. Swelling and pain returned in 90 days. Another injection followed, and another, and another. When it became obvious that surgery was the only lasting solution, to correct severe articular joint arthritis, the left knee was replaced. The same day it was replaced, I was standing and receiving help from a physical therapist. Within four months, I was again riding my horse. The replaced knee function eventually returned to 80 percent of the original normal.

Accidental dog bite

One day in 2009, I was exercising Brittany dogs with a four-wheeler all-terrain vehicle. Six dogs in sled harnesses were attached by chains to "roading bars" installed across the front and back of the machine. A seventh dog, Captain, was running free in the field beside the rest.

When I stopped to water the dogs, Captain suddenly came in from the left and attacked Sun, a rival he immensely disliked because Sun had become top dog. These two locked onto each other's throats. I managed to separate them momentarily, but Captain again lunged toward Sun, this time hitting my right hand instead of Sun's throat. It was the worst bite wound I had experienced in 52 years as a veterinarian. It left a series of noticeable scars that will last forever. Veterinarians are at high risk for bite and kick wounds, this totally unexpected bite wound happened in a blink of an eye, as true for many injuries incurred in veterinary practice.

CHAPTER 8

Finally, Classmates of the Same Grade

"I am only one, but I am still one."
– Helen Keller

School size transition

In March of 1939, after selling farm equipment and animals, we moved to the Ben Theilen farm near Maynard. Ben was Dad's uncle, and his wife, Aunt Gertie, was Grandma Theilen's sister. For the first time, I experienced riding to school on a school bus. It was a short walk of a quarter mile to the bus stop.

I went to school with my second cousins, Zola and Odell Schaller. Zola, who was older and in high school, chaperoned my first experience in a multi-roomed school. Up to that time I had been in a one-room school and always the only student in my grade. It is hard to imagine that I went through nearly five years of schooling and never had a classmate. In a sense, my early education was similar to being home-schooled, the difference being that there were other students being taught by the same teacher at different levels up to the eighth grade. Rarely were there more than 10 to 12 students at the school.

Maynard Integrated School had a student body ranging from first grade through high school. Interestingly, this was the same school my mother attended as a high school student from 1921 to 1924. While going to high school, Mom lived with the Thompson family on the north edge of Maynard. Their home was a huge two-story affair with screened porches around the top and bottom floors. Mom did housework for room and board while attending high school.

I was ahead of most of students in the fifth grade; I was slow leaner, however, in spelling and grammar. These subjects plagued me most of my educational career and early in professional life. One of my difficulties in writing occurred when I was taking "English A" in the 12th grade after we moved to Richmond, California. My English teacher became irate over a very poorly written essay. She asked "Gordon, do you plan to go to college, and where?" I replied, "Yes, UC Berkeley." As she was a recent graduate of UC Berkeley and knew that intelligence and good writing ability were necessary to succeed there, she replied: "Don't try, because you will never make it!"

Wow, those are predictive words that a teacher should never make because such comments are taken as rejection for future education. She did not know my background and my habit of never giving up on a challenge, however big it might be. This grievous comment gave me more incentive to succeed than a stern lecture ever could have done. She was putting down the Boy With the Wounded Thumb, who had made up his mind to become a veterinarian at age of 5 and needed to complete pre-veterinary studies with good grades to be accepted at a veterinary school. Later, when I became a professor at the University of California, Davis, I always remembered the put-down in high school and determined never to do the same to any of the approximately 2,700 veterinary students I taught over the years.

Yes, at times I was disappointed in the performance of some students and gave stern guidance, but I never said, "Don't try, you will never make it." I often wondered how long this teacher had a career in education. Sadly, it probably was too long.

A similar situation occurred when I recommended for acceptance to UC Davis a Hispanic student who had graduated from high school in Dixon, California, with good aptitude in math, physics, and social sciences, but poor verbal skills with low college entrance-exam scores. She had been accepted to the University of California, Santa Cruz, but as the daughter of a good and dedicated Mexican family, she wanted to attend UC Davis to be close to home to help care for a younger brother and sister; her mother and father worked every day. Her family became friends by helping us on our ranch. They had come to the United States when she was starting the eighth grade and knew no English.

I sponsored her, and she also received high regard from her school's advisor, who indicated she was of scholar quality. She was not able to speak even broken English until the ninth grade, but steadily improved academically during each of three remaining years until graduation from high school. UC Davis admissions personnel and the chancellor warned she would not make it because of poor verbal skills. I told the chancellor the story of my high school teacher's command, "Do not try, you will not make it!"

UC Davis ultimately accepted this young high school graduate, who did well. Her verbal skills did haunt her, but the combination of hard work and high IQ led her to graduate as a good student. She went on to complete a master's program at California State University, Sacramento.

Soaring like a bird

Early on a windy, stormy March day soon after we had moved to the Ben Theilen farm, a commercial tri-motored plane flew over at just tree-top level. I had a clear view of the plane making its way through a severe wind and rain storm, probably on its way from Watertown, South Dakota, to Minneapolis, about 130 miles to the east. This was a rare and memorable sight and gave a reminder of the first time I rode in an open-cockpit plane, at the Chippewa County Fair in 1938. I had begged my mother to ride with me in a biplane. We almost didn't go for the ride. As my mother was purchasing tickets, a man came up to her and said, "Missus, I would not go for a ride in that rattletrap; it had to make an emergency landing yesterday in a nearby farm field." My mother wanted to back out, but I begged her to stick with what was a first flying experience for both of us.

The flight was an amazing experience for a 10-year-old who loved the unexpected. I was fascinated to view the Earth a few thousand feet below: I was soaring like a pigeon, a robin, or a blackbird. I had not seen an eagle soar, but I observed many small birds flying freely above the Earth and going from limb to limb in trees with unquestionable ease.

From the air, I saw the confluence of the Minnesota and Chippewa rivers where I swam in a way previously unimaginable. It was fascinating to see how the rivers meandered through the country that I knew well from bicycling in the same area. We flew from Montevideo to Granite Falls, and saw falls on the Minnesota River. Wow – it was an experience that vastly differed from viewing them just a few hundred feet away from the banks of the river. We could not hear the roar of the falls; the plane's engines made so much noise that Mom and I could not even hear each other speak.

I did not go up in a plane again until jump-school training for the paratroopers in 1946, a turn of events that I had not anticipated eight years before. I had to be fearless of heights and have feeling of security that the attached break-away cord in the C-46 aircraft would pull the chute open as I fell 90 feet out of the plane going 120 miles an hour. Again, I reveled in seeing the wonders of the Earth from 1,000 feet above ground level.

Family misunderstanding

In May of 1939 there was an imbroglio with the Ben Theilen family, who had no children, considered Dad as their son, and wanted him to farm their land. The farm eventually was to become our farm. Ben and Gera (Gertie) made initial arrangements to move to town. However, they decided to stay on the farm and shared the house with our family. It was crowded to say the least. The Ben Theilen farm was only 180 acres and would not support a family of four and two retired relatives. The somewhat rolling terrain was less than ideal farm land. Ben was Dad father's brother, and Gertie was Dad mother's sister. Dad's sister Gera (Gertie) was named after her aunt, Gertie Theilen.

The house had not been properly cleaned for several years and needed scouring. My mother was dedicated to keeping a clean house and wanted years of waste on the floors to be scrubbed away, especially in the kitchen and dining area. For some unknown reason, Uncle Ben probably thought this cleaning was an affront to his wife. He became irate with my mother. Ben began to yell and then threaten my mother with physical violence. She immediately contacted Dad, who was doing field work, and he without hesitation decided to leave immediately. This was the final straw that initiated an eventual move to the West.

Travel westward

We lived for a short time with my mom's parents north of Maynard, where I finished the last few days of school. In mid-June, I went to Le Mars, Iowa, to spend time with my Iowa relatives. I felt important living in a block-square area with a huge courthouse and county jail with living quarters for the family. My parents, along with my sister, Blythe, were to arrive in two weeks, but my mother became ill with a kidney infection (Bright's disease) and our trip to the West coast was postponed for six weeks. In August the trip began, the four of us traveling in a 1933 Plymouth two-door sedan with a travel trunk attached to the rear. All clothes, cookware, and some food items were packed into the trunk. Motels in those days provided facilities to cook meals. We looked much like the nomadic families in John Steinbeck's classic novel *The Grapes of Wrath*.

Dad, having traveled to the West Coast in 1922, followed the route he had taken then along with his brother, Ben, Mom's brother, Charlie, John Thompson and Ralph Blakesley, who were from Minnesota, and Uncle Ben from Iowa. We left Le Mars, Iowa, and traveled through Nebraska, past the Devil's Tower, a geological landmark, now a national monument. It was interesting to see the western edge of the plains meet the eastern slope of the Rocky Mountains in Wyoming. As we traveled U.S. 40, the Lincoln Highway, alongside the Green River, we went from lower elevation and steadily gained altitude to the summit at around 7,000 feet, all within one day.

Dad was on pins and needles as the old 1933 Plymouth heated up, but he took the grade slowly and the radiator did not boil over. I had my photo taken with a Sioux Indian chief at one of the stops in Wyoming. This was my first opportunity to see real Indians, and even at 12 years old I was cautious, remembering stories that my grandmother Theilen told me. When she grew up on the farm in western Iowa in the 1870s, Indians were considered marauders and nomads.

Dad had been fascinated by the Mormon Tabernacle complex in Salt Lake City, Utah, in his 1920 visit and a return visit in 1922. It was somewhat of an attempt to become better acquainted with Mormonism. The visit to the Tabernacle (an assembly hall open to the public) was the first instruction I had ever had with acoustics. The Tabernacle interior is so sonically resonant that a pin being dropped into a hat can be heard many feet away. The architecture of the Temple, the sanctuary that is restricted to devout, upper-level Mormons, gave an impression of "beware: off limits!" I had never experienced "off limits" at any churches I had attended or seen up to that time. The monument in the center of Temple Square was of a seagull. It was that species of bird that saved the harvest of the early settlers in this area of Utah.

We swam in the Great Salt Lake, and what an experience – it was impossible to sink due to the high salinity of the water. My mother was fearful to go in since she could not swim, yet she did wade in a short distance from shore. I had the experience of swimming in the Dead Sea in 1990 and again experienced the sensation of inability to sink in salinized water.

While crossing Nevada, we saw snow plows that were used to move billions of crickets off old Highway 40. This was the same type of infestation that Mormon settlers had experienced many years earlier in the western Utah area of their settling journey westward. In that locust plague millions of seagulls arrived to devour the billions of insects that destroyed their crops.

We also visited Reno, "biggest little city in the world." I had never been exposed to public gambling and so many blinking neon lights. We stayed in Reno one night. Mom allowed me to put a nickel in a slot machine and – guess what? – I lost the nickel.

We had to ascend the Sierra Nevada, going from 4,500 feet elevation at Reno to Donner Summit at 7,057 feet. Dad told us about the plight of the Donner Party of pioneers who were stranded by snow in 1849, and how the awful time they had prompted some desperate members of the group to resort to cannibalism to stay alive. They spent the winter at 6,000 feet and finally were rescued in late April. The snowfall that year was horrendous, battering the mountains with storm after storm.

As we descended the western slope of the Sierra to Auburn, we encountered unbearable heat. The temperature was 100 degrees and increased as we approached Sacramento, where the thermometer read 114. It stayed that hot as we traveled on the three-lane Yolo causeway crossing and drive through every town, including Davis, which I later would call home for 40 years.

We continued through Dixon, Vacaville, and Fairfield, all in unrelenting heat. Then we started up the Coast Range grade to go through Vallejo and cross the three-lane bridge over the Carquinez Strait. At this point we were fascinated by low-lying clouds, which turned out to be fog. The breeze was blowing at a cool temperature off San Pablo Bay. We drove through Rodeo, then along the bay in fog to Hercules, where Dad would eventually work for 25 years. We drove through Pinole and descended down the three-lane Tank Farm Hill grade to a motel on the northern edge of San Pablo. This was at the base of Tank Farm Hill (so named for a complex of Standard Oil of California storage tanks).

It was about dark when we arrived there and the temperature was 55 degrees with a strong westerly wind off the San Pablo Bay. We checked into a motel on San Pablo Avenue. When taking things from the trunk into the motel, the first thing we noticed was how warm everything was in the trunk and how cool it was outside. We had difficulty reconciling the fact that it was summer, yet the temperature was 55 degrees and we needed to use the motel-room heater for warmth. We soon learned that our first encounter with the cool, foggy summer weather was not an aberration, but rather was the norm for the San Francisco Bay Area in summer.

A miracle at Treasure Island

We arrived in California in time to see the 1939–1940 Golden Gate International Exposition at Treasure Island in San Francisco Bay. My Dad had not intended to remain in the San Francisco Bay Area, but rather to continue northward to Seattle, where his brother, Ben, had a job for him at Sand Point Naval Shipyard. My mother was leery of living near and around Ben's wife, Louise, whom she had met on a visit to Minnesota shortly after Ben and Louise were married in 1937. Mom had a very cautious feeling about her.

The Lord leads often in mysterious ways, and lives change instantaneously as a result of His guidance. On an August Saturday afternoon at the Golden Gate Exposition, my sister, Blythe, became temporarily lost. Over the loudspeaker system we heard an announcement: "A little girl by the name of Blythe is looking for her parents, and she is at the Lutheran Hour Booth." That was a group that broadcast Sunday morning Lutheran worship services on the radio.

People at the booth were interested to learn that we were Lutherans from Minnesota and on our way to Washington to live. They invited us to attend Trinity Lutheran Church the next day. It was located about 15 city blocks from the motel where we were staying. Pastor Otto Rohrer was the minister, and after services he greeted us at the door with his wife, Lillian.

Obvious questions were asked. Why were we in Richmond? Dad indicated we would be on our way the next day to Seattle, where his brother, Ben, lived and was going to help Dad get a job. The pastor indicated that jobs were available in Richmond. Why not stay a few additional days and consider living in Richmond?

"Lillian and our two kids and I are going on vacation tomorrow, and you can stay in the parsonage while we are gone and decide whether you wish to live in Richmond," he told us. My parents agreed, and we relocated to the parsonage. Within a few days a member of the congregation, Mr. Kerber, had arranged for Dad to start a job at an American Standard factory where porcelain toilets and sinks were made. When Pastor Rohrer and his family returned, the house was spick and span from house cleaning, and apple pies were awaiting them.

The Theilen family in the meantime had rented a one-bedroom apartment owned by the McCouley family on Barrett between 21st and 20th streets. We started life in Richmond in August 1939. Dad would die in Richmond from a heart attack in April 1965, and never again returned to the cold winters in Minnesota and sharecrop farming.

The Lord led the family to set new roots where the Boy With the Wounded Thumb eventually would follow his desire to become a veterinarian. It was a substantial change, as I was used to farm life and now lived in a one-bedroom apartment with no animals around. I had to find new friends, and play on cement sidewalks and asphalt streets. Few friends lived on a small farm in outskirts of Richmond, and those few lived at least a mile away. In Richmond, friends lived across the street, including the McCouleys' grandson, Ralph Pinchon. He was the leader of the neighborhood gang until we had a fistfight that I won by hitting him so hard it broke his nose. This unfortunate fight resulted not in becoming enemies but rather dear friends with tremendous respect for each other. This was one few fist fights in which I was involved. After that, I utilized diplomacy and subdued aggression the rest of my life.

CHAPTER 9

The Beginning of New Experiences in Richmond

"My life is spent in one long effort to escape from the commonplace of existence."

— Sherlock Holmes

Richmond in 1939 was a city of 15,000 people for the most part settled after the San Francisco earthquake of 1906. That disaster depopulated San Francisco, sending many residents to the East Bay. Point Richmond was the original settlement in what was to become a much larger city, spreading to the east over former agricultural lands.

The main street west to east was MacDonald Avenue, center of the business district. In 1939, the city was mainly lower to middle-middle class. The upper-middle class lived east of San Pablo Avenue, which extended from the small town of San Pablo to Oakland. Barrett Avenue extended from First Street to the top of Mira Vista Hills east of San Pablo. This was an area of expensive homes, and some people living there were wealthy. The less fortunate lived in North Richmond, located a mile north of downtown and extending along Tenth Street. Most people there were of dark-skinned ethnicity. Most kids from the entire city went to Richmond Unified High School.

As we settled for a future life in Richmond. I learned to love the cool summer weather. Now, having lived 65 years in the Sacramento Valley communities of Davis and Dixon, I cope with the daytime heat, and relish the cool Delta breezes in most summer evenings, when temperatures soothingly drop into the 60s. What a wonderful feeling! The Pacific Ocean not far away is a natural air conditioner designed by God.

Sixth grade: One room, 30 students

August 1939 quickly sped away until it was time for my sister, Blythe, and me to start school. The Theilen family lived at the Barrett Avenue Apartments on the first floor of a four-unit building. There were plenty of playmates.

Sixth grade began at Grant Grammar School. There were 25 children in sixth grade. I established what would become lifelong friendships with several classmates, including Dick Macfie, Ron Kamb, Dick McGranahan, Ray Moitosa, Bob Feenan, Elaine Robertson and others. Elaine sat across the aisle from me, and I remembered her as a mathematical star. Remember, this was the first time the Boy With the Wounded Thumb was in a classroom devoted entirely to a single grade. I was ahead of other students in most subjects at Grant School, but lingered behind in spelling, English, writing, and penmanship. I excelled early in most other subjects, particularly those relating to biology and physical sciences.

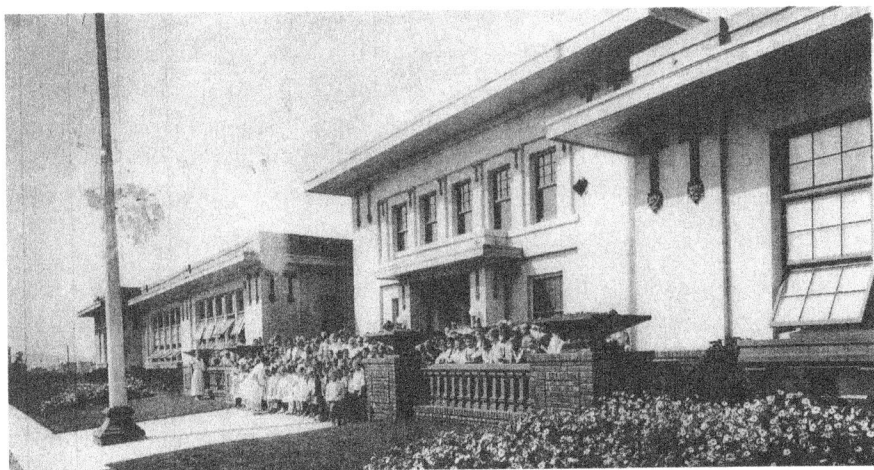

Grant School on Grant Avenue in Richmond, with students in front (Compliments of Ron Kamb, classmate from 1939).

My friends and I spent recesses playing kickball, pole ball, hopscotch, and tag. The fifth-grade teacher, Miss Neukom, was a terror if a pupil became rowdy during recess. She would routinely pull ears, slap the back of a rowdy student's hands with a ruler, and sometimes give them a swat on the butt. Miss Elliott, the sixth-grade teacher, seemed to have an easier manner with pupils. I remember her favorably, along with my first- to third-grade teacher, Amy Anderson.

The Goen brothers, Lyle and Cecil, were part of the gang who lived on Barrett near 20th Street. We started playing sandlot football, tackling and all, with no protective gear. We would pretend that we were famous football stars along the lines of George Gipp, a.k.a. "the Gipper," whom Ronald Reagan played in *Knute Rockne, All American,* a 1940 biographical Hollywood movie about Notre Dame football. We also tried to imitate Red Grange, a famous University of Illinois player, and many other famous players (especially, for me, players from the University of Minnesota, coached under Bernie Bierman). Neighborhood six-man touch football teams organized through the Richmond Recreational Department practiced after school and played teams from other grammar schools on Saturday mornings September through November.

In the fall, the Richmond Recreational Department provided for several six-man touch football teams based at various grammar schools. At Grant Grammar School, I was part of a touch football team, the members of which included Ralph Pinchon, Dick Macfie, Bob Feenan, and Ray Moitosa. That paved the way for me to became a lifelong football fan. I remember the young female adviser who taught the young kids to block and run. Play was stopped by tagging the runner with the ball (tag football). The young UC Berkeley co-ed took the team to a football game at Memorial Stadium on the campus one fall Saturday afternoon. Cal played U of Washington that day, and I vividly remember one of their players being severely injured and taken off the field on a stretcher. It turned out to be a bad back injury and broken vertebrae in the neck.

Being in a stadium with 40,000 people cheering for their team or against the opposing team was a new and extremely exciting experience. When the game was over, students sang "Hail to California." Seven decades later, the Boy With the Wounded Thumb still remembers the feeling of pride that swept the stadium. On that day in 1939, however, I did not realize that I would attend UC Berkeley 10 years later as a pre-veterinary student. Wow, how coincidental events in one's life are miracles of recall!

CHAPTER 10

Encephalomyelitis – Comatosing Illness

"He loves nature in spite of what it did to him."
– Forrest Tucker

Fall became winter. Sometime in December 1939, I was ill with a fever of 107 Fahrenheit and slipped into a coma. In an era before sulfa and antibiotic drugs, Dr. Geinen ordered slow-drip IV fluids and oxygen. On the third day of my hospitalization, when I remained comatose with a consistent fever of 107, the doctor indicated to my parents that they should inform relatives in Minnesota and Iowa that I was not expected to live through the night. But about 4 o'clock the next morning, the fever started coming down. In a sweat, I was on the road to slow recovery.

A definitive diagnosis was not made, but Dr. Geinen suggested that it probably was a case of encephelospinal meningitis. I was weak from the illness for several weeks after hospitalization. I did not attend school again until January. The family moved to a house on 18th Street near Esmond Avenue during my recovery.

Scourge of poison oak dermatitis

About eight weeks after hospitalization I felt good enough to go to San Pablo Creek, and there I was exposed to poison oak for the first time, leading to severe

61

contact dermatitis. The plant alkaloid caused my skin to become inflamed and itchy, and when I scratched it, a bacterial infection attacked the abraded tissue. I looked like a balloon and itched all over. Bright pink calamine lotion helped to ease the itching.

I was in an immune-compromised state from the previous illness, and after the sores started to heal I became infested with boils. The boils were caused by the bacterial staphylococcus infection that resulted from scratching. Aggravated by my temporary low immunity to subcutaneous-induced infections, the boils progressed to unbelievable large abscesses. Multiple boils persisted, and after one would burst with purulent exudate, others would develop. Mom placed bread poultices soaked in milk over each sore, along with hot Epsom salt (magnesium sulfate) compresses. New boils developed for several months, most prominently on my waistline, arms, thighs, and legs. I have a multitude of scars from healed abscesses as this book is written.

Hives

After the bout with boils, I became afflicted with hives (skin allergic eruptions all over the body) that itched and were slightly painful. These persisted for two to three months. As a 12-year-old, I went to Dr. Geinen on my own, because Mom and Dad were working full time – Dad at Hercules Powder Company and Mom at a fish cannery along San Pablo Bay in North Richmond. Dr. Geinen gave me hemotherapy by withdrawing 20cc of blood from the radial artery of my arm and immediately injecting it into thigh muscle at several locations. I underwent a second hemotherapy treatment 10 days later. The hives totally disappeared and have never returned. This miraculous recovery resulted from stimulating stem cells to initiate an immune response. I have used immunotherapy in treating cancer, as my book *One Medicine War on Cancer* will describe.

In the 1940s, doctors, veterinarians, and other professionals did not worry about lawsuits as they do in the 21st century. I often wonder if we are destroying ourselves as a culture by employing too many lawyers. Since the 1940 hives episode I have experienced hives after touching short-haired dogs, mostly of German breed origin, such as Doberman pinchers, boxers, and dachshunds. The hives came on suddenly and quickly. The good news was they also quickly went away, lasting only a few hours.

Liberty Magazines and community honesty

During the months of recovery from encephalomyelitis, I began to sell *Liberty* magazines for five cents a copy with two cents profit. *Liberty* was a weekly, general-interest magazine popular at the time. I hired the Goen brothers to sell for me, and they got a penny, as did I, for each copy they sold. I used the money I earned to buy a bicycle, and rode it to see movies during Saturday matinees at the Fox Theater on MacDonald Avenue between Ninth and Tenth streets on the north side. Bicycles were not locked, and no one in 1940 would think of stealing one, in front of a theater or any other place. Our homes at 18th Street and at 28th and Gaynor were never locked. Richmond then was safe, relatively thief-proof. It deteriorated in the 1960s, becoming largely a ghetto in certain areas. Downtown became unsafe to walk, and no one would leave a bicycle unlocked anywhere from then on.

Our own home

In 1940 my parents purchased a lot on 28th at Gaynor and built a house on the southwest corner. It was a three-bedroom, one-bath house with an unattached two-car garage. Dad had worked with his father, who was a carpenter, and knew about carpentry. With the help of a contractor, Mr. Christiansen, they built our home. We moved in near the end of the year. It was the first owned home for my parents, and the furniture was all new. The area was semirural; Gaynor had a sidewalk, but 28th did not. A block north on Esmond Avenue, residents still had chickens, cows, goats, and pigs.

1941: Newspaper delivery

I began to work at age 13 in 1941 by delivering newspapers – first the *Oakland Post-Enquirer,* an afternoon paper, and then the *Richmond Record,* a morning publication. The afternoon paper route started after school and was in and around 23rd Street from MacDonald Avenue to Esmond Avenue in the north. The morning paper route started at 6 a.m. was delivered from 23rd Street to the south of MacDonald all the way to First Street.

The Kaiser Shipyards were in full swing, and while I was delivering morning papers before dawn, the sound of riveting filled the air, and lights from the yards lit up areas south of MacDonald like it was dawn. The song "Rosie the Riveter," about a woman who helped construct Liberty ships at the yard, became a national hit, and Rosie became a national icon and symbol of feminism. There is a Rosie the Riveter Museum now at the location of the shipyard she worked. With amazing speed, workers built Victory and Liberty cargo ships, which were absolutely necessary to transport cargo from the mainland to the Pacific Theater for fighting the Japanese, and to England in readying for the invasion of France at Normandy on June 6, 1944.

I would arise at 3:30 a.m. and make breakfast, almost always fried cornmeal drenched in Karo syrup, along with a cup of coffee. Off I would go from 28th and Gaynor about a mile to 23rd and MacDonald, to obtain morning papers at the Richmond Record printing shop.

Vienna Bakery

A year later, work for me began at 4 a.m. one morning and 5 a.m. the next for six days a week at the Vienna Bakery on the west side of 23rd Street, just before MacDonald Avenue. It was near the newspaper print shop. Lyle Goen worked there as well. We would fry donuts in hot grease vats and then glaze them. I ate so many donuts that it was literally 40 years later before I again ate one. One morning, Lyle stepped into a five-gallon pail of chocolate pudding intended for chocolate éclairs. His shoe filled with the mix. He took it off and tipped the pudding back into the pail. What we often don't know when we eat at a restaurant or purchase goods from a bakery!

Junior high, 1940–1943

My memory of Longfellow Junior High School at 23rd and Nevin Avenue is sketchy, as school time was only half-days. Roosevelt Junior High was closed at the time. Something had happened to the facilities, and all of that school's students shared space at Longfellow. I was so busy with paper routes, working in the bakery, and doing other things that I don't remember much about school. I do, however, remember wood shop class and the ash-tray stand I built for Dad. He used it as a place for his pipe every day until he died. The octagon-shaped top with four legs is now more than 75 years old. When my mother sold her personal belongings at an estate sale, she saved the stand for me. It is now in my office. Mr. Doss Thompson, the woodshop teacher, was extremely helpful. Presently, several times a day I see the small wood stand next to my desk; for a fleeting moment I remember Longfellow Junior High, the years of puberty, and finding my way to gain my dream of becoming a veterinarian.

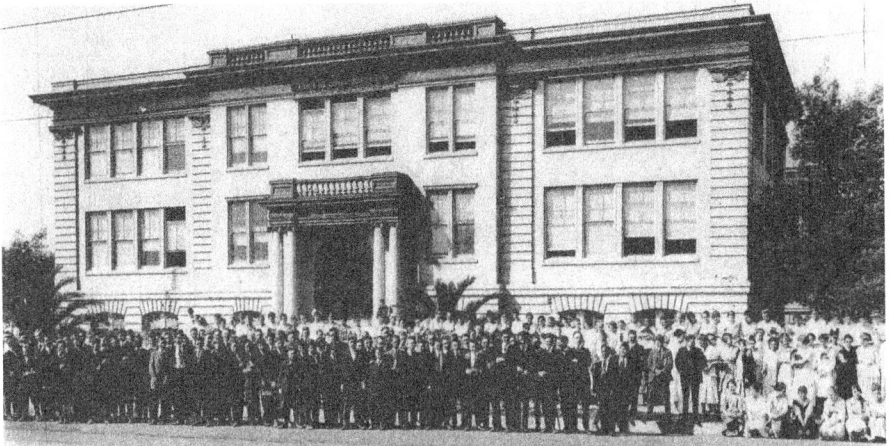

Longfellow Junior High on 23rd and Nevin streets, Richmond, California. Compliments of Ron Kamb, classmate in the graduating class of 1942.

Another remembrance of junior high was gym class. Mr. Frank Bagnes was the gym coach. When he was teaching us and discussing some aspects of the class at the beginning of the year, I was not paying attention and disturbed the class by horsing around. He came over and shook me until he ripped the new sweat jersey that I'd had to purchase for the class.

After delivering afternoon newspapers, I went home to find Dad. I told him what happened and asked him to go to the school principal and tell him about the cruel way the teacher had treated me. Dad asked, "Gordon what did you do to have him act the way he did?" I told dad the truth and he replied, "If you had paid attention, this would not have happened. I expect you to become a more attentive student in the future." This was a lesson well taught, and since Dad did not overreact about school discipline, I never again approached my parents about sticking up for me at school over a matter of discipline I deserved.

Christian confirmation

In addition to being busy with paper routes and work in the bakery, I also attended after-school confirmation classes at Trinity Lutheran Church. I was confirmed in April 1942 in a class of five, the other members of which were Loraine Kerber, Walter and Bob Furst, and a girl whose name I do not remember. I was always close to the Lord, and teachings by Pastor Otto Rohrer brought me closer. Pastor Rohrer was a convert from Roman Catholicism and

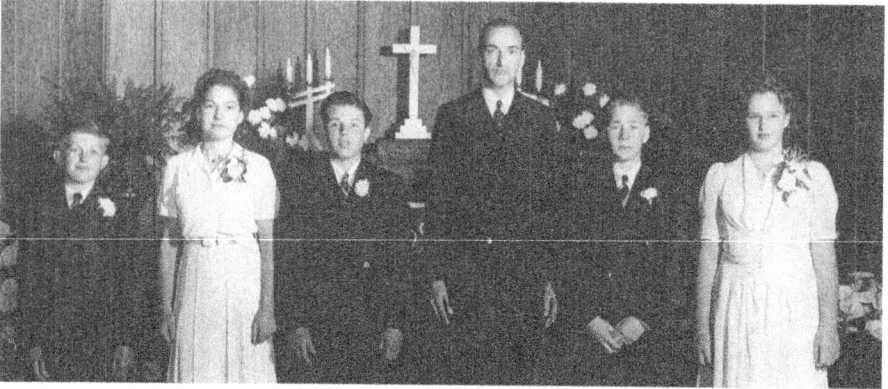

Confirmation with Pastor Rohrer and fellow students.

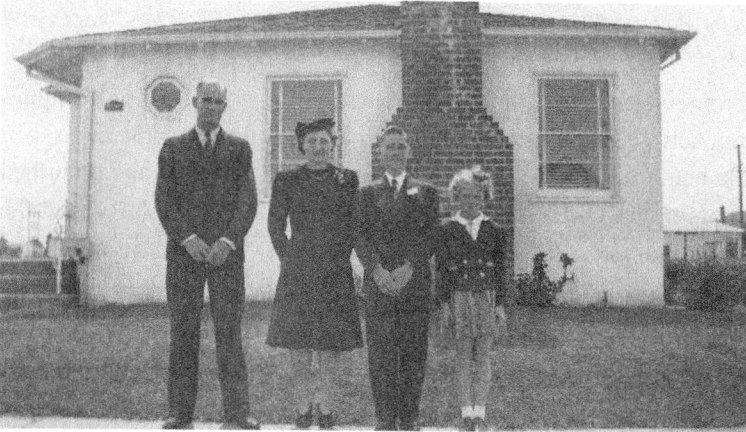

Me with my parents and Blythe in front of our new home at 2750 Gaynor on confirmation day.

held Luther's major Christian tenets very dear to his newfound understanding of the Holy Scriptures. Faith alone, Grace alone and The Word alone were the main emphasis, then as now, in Christian Lutheranism. You are saved by the grace of God, not by doing good works, and show thanks by studying His Word and keeping the Christian faith.

Junior high friendship

David Flagg and I were bicycling at Point Richmond one very warm Sunday morning – December 7, 1941. We stopped for a soft drink at a roadside refreshment stand on Cutting Boulevard and received the news that the Japanese had attached Pearl Harbor. David was horrified, because his father was in the way of danger. That day changed our lives for many years. David's father was a civilian worker at Wake Island who was captured when the Japanese invaded. Mr. Flagg was sent to a prisoner-of-war camp in Shanghai, where he remained until his release when the Japanese surrendered in 1945.

David and I became good friends. He had musical talent and a great interest in world affairs. He was an avid outdoors person and fortunate to have grandparents who lived in Potter Valley, near Ukiah. He and I spent a holiday break in the winter of 1942 with his grandparents. We boys had a marvelous time in the outdoors, and I shot my first deer, out of season, but it was wartime and our family consumed the venison. All citizens were on food rationing, meat was limited, and I was proud to bring meat to the family dinner table.

David lived on 22nd Street and would list the city names of each of the Greyhound buses that stopped at the nearby 23rd Street bus station. In those days each Greyhound bus had the name of an American city, such as Denver, Omaha, Salt Lake City, and so forth, including ones rarely seen, such as Sioux Falls.

David's mother used to work in a soda fountain on MacDonald near the Fox Theater. We had a three-tiered ice cream cone for the cost of a one-scoop, five-cent cone due to his mother's influence. David and I traveled all over town on bicycles and often went to a large indoor swimming pool just off Cutting Boulevard in Point Richmond. It was the only municipal swimming pool in town at the time.

David and I would give a report daily in history class about the latest international happenings with the German armies sweeping through France and other countries. The two of us kept track of newspaper accounts of what was happening in Europe, Asia, and North and South America. No other students seemed to be so interested in the battles of World War II.

When it came time for David to start high school in 1943, his mother sent him to military academy. The strong friendship never again was able to surface. Many years later, David and his wife contacted us at our Linden Lane address in Davis, California. David had become a gospel singer and recorded many Christian hymns. We lost contact in the 1970s, and I have no idea what happened during those years; I learned that David died on March 27, 2016, in Orinda, California. We were exceptionally good boyhood friends.

CHAPTER 11

1942: Summer in Iowa and Minnesota

"What we have once enjoyed we can never lose;
all that we love deeply becomes a part of us."
– Helen Keller

In the summer of 1942 I traveled by train, as a 14-year-old, to spend my vacation in Iowa and Minnesota with relatives. Money for the trip came from my work as a newspaper boy and bakery helper. I occupied a chair seat from Richmond all the way to Le Mars, Iowa, and then to Maynard, Minnesota. A young sailor on leave who had the adjoining seat was my chaperone to Omaha, where I transferred to Sioux City and then to Le Mars.

Le Mars

Aunt Emma and Uncle Frank Scholer met me at the train station. Darrel and Bud, first cousins of mine, were working in Sioux City at the construction site for the military air base being built for the World War II effort. This meant that they were gone from early in the morning until late at night, and I was on my own to go swimming at White Way Sand Pit. My dad as a youngster swam there from 1910 to 1916. I would ride Bud's bicycle to the swimming hole, fondly remember Le Mars, as it was a time to be with beloved Iowa relatives.

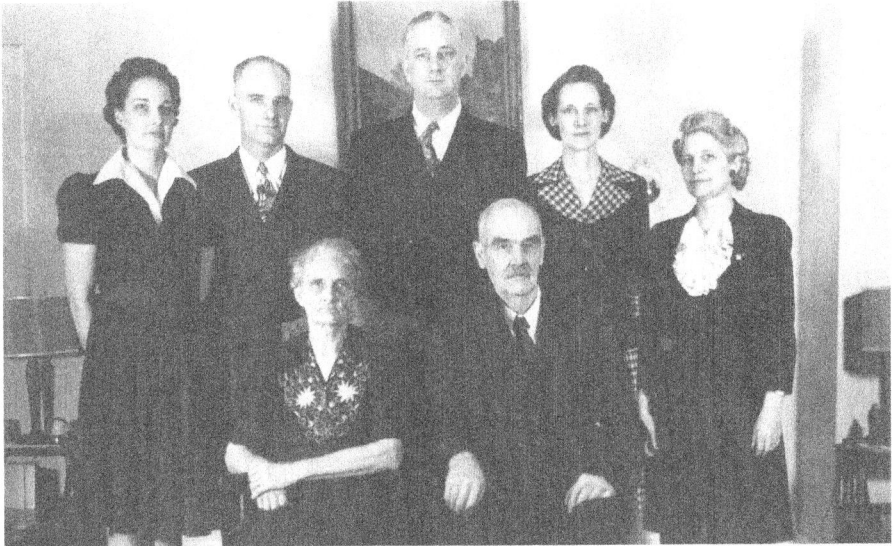

Grandparent Meta and Henry Theilen celebrating their 50th anniversary with their five children: Marjorie, Lou (Dad), Ben, Gera (Gertie) and Emma.

I had visits with Grandma and Grandpa Theilen, who sat on their porch most summer evenings, slowly swinging back and forth. They mostly communicated in silence. Their parents were from Ostfriesland (East Friesland), near the Dutch border in Northern Germany. The Ostfrieslanders are tall people; men are often over six feet tall. My grandfather stood six feet eight inches tall, and grandmother six feet.

People from Ostfriesland have a culture of few words. Grandpa smoked a pipe and was a retired carpenter. In 1942 he enjoyed gardening and keeping bees. My grandparents lost their life savings in the stock market crash of 1929 and the closing of banks in the early days of the Roosevelt administration. A similar scenario occurred some 80 years later with the huge monetary crash of October 2008. Many people lost their life savings and jobs in 2008, and four years later finding employment remained difficult. There is a cyclical pattern to economic ups and downs, but such conditions could not have been worse for Henry and Meta (Grandma) Theilen. After the crash of 1929, they never regained a middle-class standard of living. They were poor and survived mainly by gardening and canning.

I remember eating ice-cream cones at a stand on Center Street. The stand was supplied by Wells Dairy, a hometown business that since has become

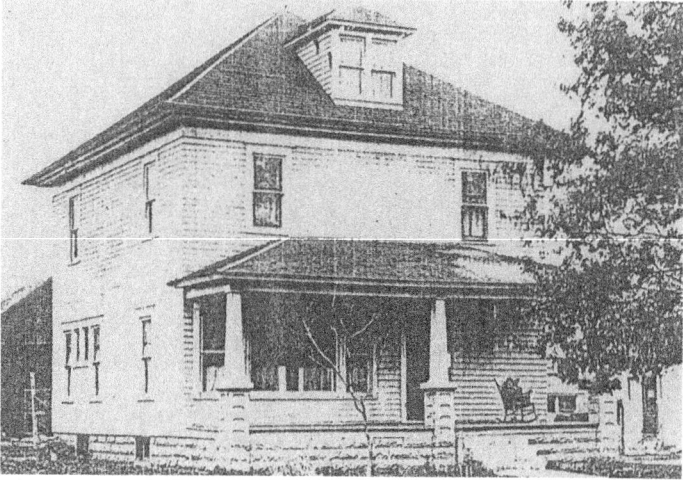

The Theilen home that Grandpa built.]

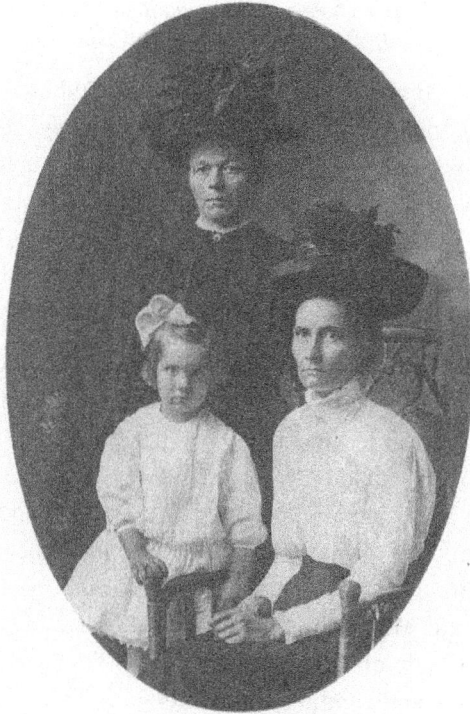

Great grandmother Anke Collmann, Grandmother Meta, and Aunt Gera,(Gertie) who was 6 years old when this photo was taken in 1909.

70

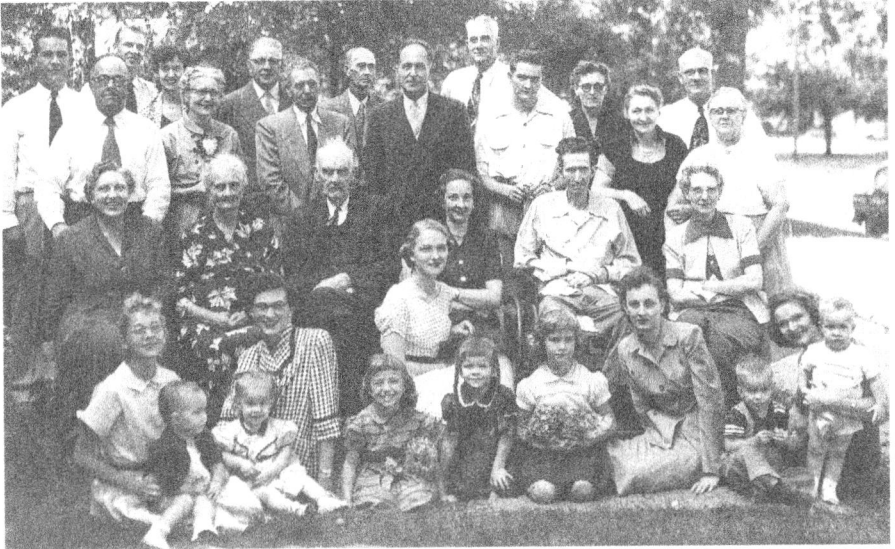

This Theilen family photo shows my grandparents celebrating their 50th anniversary, in the company their five children, Ema Theilen and my sister, Blythe, and other family members.

the nation's largest family-owned distributor of ice cream products. Recently the Wells Creamery was sold to a national syndicated firm. I would go to the ice cream stand with cousins Janet Juhle and her sister, Brenda, who was a little girl in 1942. I frequently saw Dad's youngest sister, Margorie (Sidy), her husband Alex, who had multiple sclerosis, their son James, and daughter, Judy. Sidy was caretaker for Alex, who was a paraplegic. She worked as secretary at the local livestock auction yard. Dad's three sisters lived in Le Mars until Sidy and Alex moved to Cherokee, where Sidy lived until she was in advanced age. Both aunts, Emma and Sidy, developed Alzheimer's disease. Emma lived to be 101 and Sidy to 99. Sidy fondly remembered into her early 90s that she was one of my Baptismal sponsors. The other sponsor was my grandfather Henry Schaller. Emma and Frank took me out to dinner occasionally at a restaurant where I always ordered a beef and jack sandwich on white bread topped with a creamy white gravy. Ema and Frank treated me as well as a son.

Maynard

Later in July, I traveled from Remsen near Le Mars for a direct train to Maynard. The train stopped at every town along with way, so that 200-mile journey took eight hours. I spent the next several weeks with Grandpa and Grandma Schaller (Henry and Amelia, referred to as "Millie"), who met me at the train station. Henry (Hank) had recently retired from farming due to severe leg problems following a botched surgical procedure to treat a prostate problem. Grandma helped Aunt Fern with the housework, milked a few cows, and fed farm animals. They lived with Harold and Fern Sulflow. Harold had been a farmhand, married Fern, and eventually became owner of the farm. I was reintroduced to farming and doing odd jobs. However, Harold Sulflow was difficult to please, never satisfied with my endeavors. I helped in small ways. I became good friends with Harold Tebben, a high-school student and distant cousin who worked for Harold Sulflow.

My grandfather Henry Schaller was born in Schneckenlohe, Germany, Northern Bavaria, in the area of ueber Franken (above Franken), or north of the location referred to as Franken. Schnekenlohe was a small village in forested, rolling hills and moderately high mountains not far from Coburg and the neighboring province of Sacheny. His home and farm were on Friedhof Strasse, the cemetery street, about a kilometer from the graveyard, on property that has been owned by the Schaller family since the 17th century.

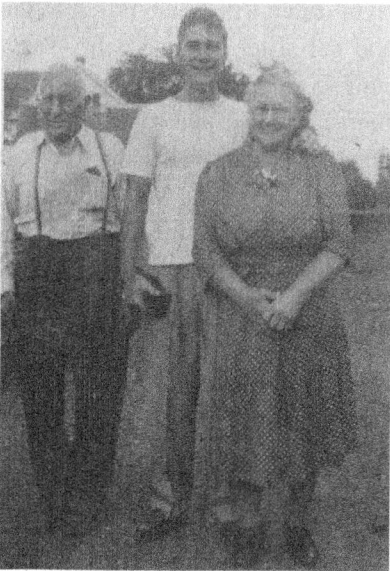

My Schaller grandparents with me during a 1942 visit.

My ancestors migrated to that community around 1640 and their descendents have lived on the same farm since. Villages since the reformation and up to the present are Roman Catholic (Katholisch) or Lutheran (Evangalisch) residents. Schnekenlohe is a Roman Catholic village. The Schallers, being Lutheran, went to the Lutheran Church in Schmoltz, five kilometers east of Schneckenlohe. At that Lutheran church, a pastor baptized and confirmed them, and performed marriage and burial ceremonies for them.

Hank (Grandfather's nickname) first came to the United States as a 15-year-old, with two younger brothers, Karl

72

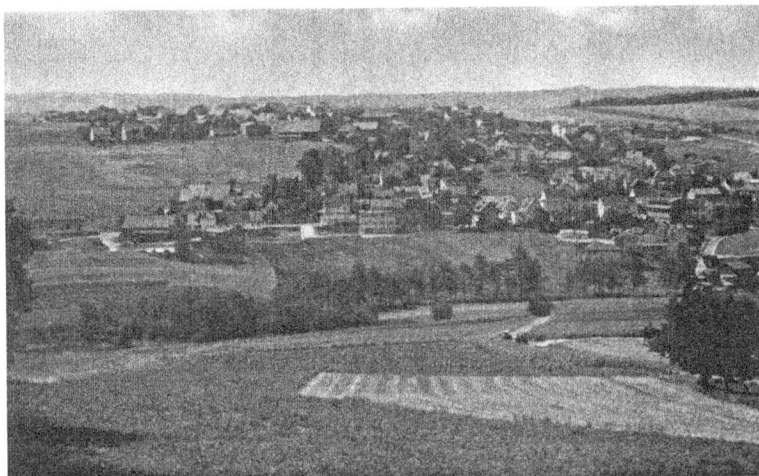

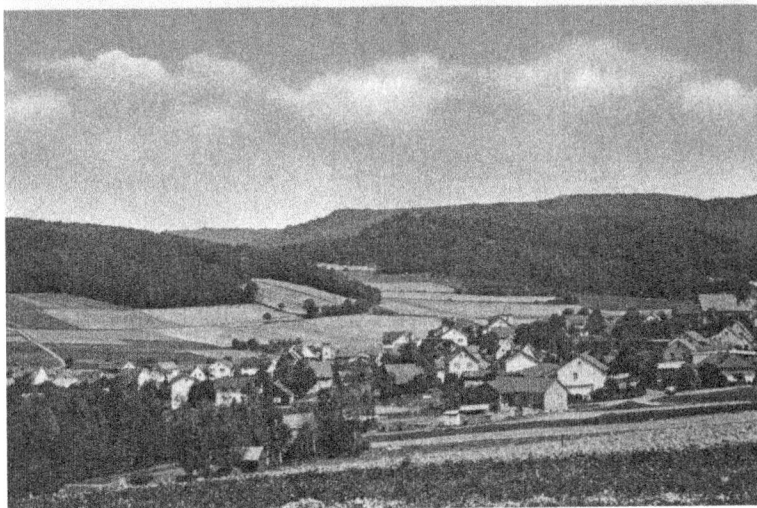

A postcard showing the village where Grandpa Schaller grew up. The property is on the east side of Schneckenlohe on Friedhof Strasse.

(Charles) and Emile. They came through Ellis Island and immigrated to Sterling, Illinois, where Hank was father and brother to Charles and Emile. As a single parent, he worked in a wire mill for less than a dollar a day with 12-hour shifts, six days a week. When Hank was 20, he returned to Germany to visit family members and while there, he was conscripted into the German Army for two years. He had not yet become an American citizen, and all German men served at least two years in the military.

After discharge, Hank returned to America with his younger sister, Anna. The entire family eventually moved to Minnesota and farmed in the Maynard area on former swamp land that had been drained for agricultural use. Hank lived three miles north of town, and Charles two miles east. Anna (Annie) married twice. Her first husband, Mr. Aldis Harting, died after a relatively short marriage. They had three children. Her second marriage was to Mr. Chris Hemingsen. Chris had been married previously with 3 children. The couple lived near Redwood Falls, about 30 miles from the two brothers, Hank and Charlie. Emile settled in the Greenbush area near the Canadian border. The three brothers and sister never became rich, but they always provided for their families and never worked for others.

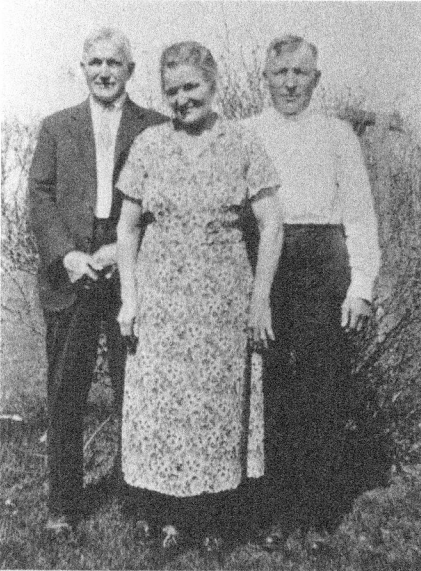

Uncle Charles (at left), Aunt Annie Hemingsen, and Grandpa Schaller.

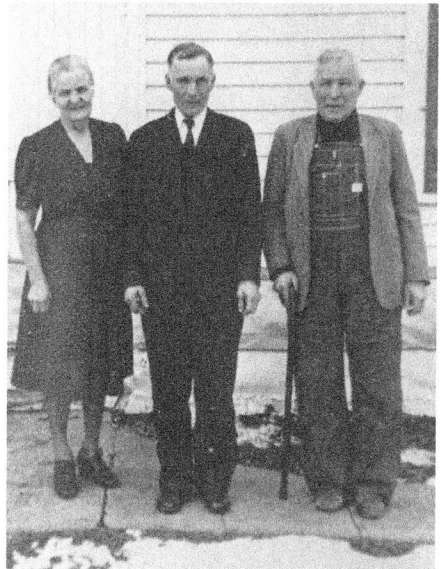

Aunt Annie (left), Uncle Emile Schaller, and Grandpa.

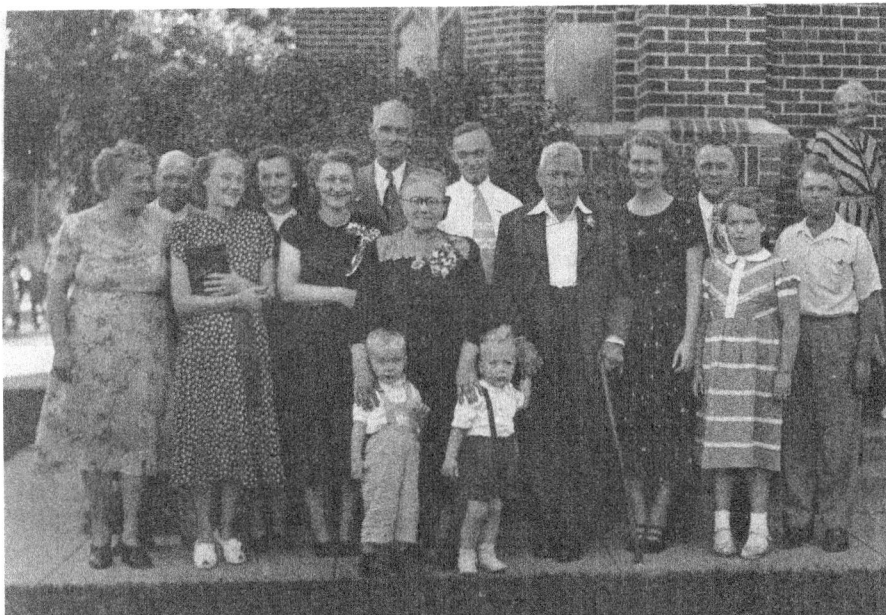

[My Schaller grandparents celebrating their 50th wedding anniversary with four living children, spouses and young grandchildren.]

Year 800 to present:
L'Epagneul Breton and Western Europe

Franken is the area where Karl the Grosser and his army originated. From there, his army went westward, crossing the River Main at what later became known as Frankfurt (crossing of the Franks). He continued on to conquer Gaul, much territory of which France now occupies. France got its name from the Franks; in local language the "k" was dropped and "ce" added in its place. Karl the Grosser is known in France as a founding father, affectionately called Charlemagne (the "main" or great Charles). Charlemagne conquered most of Western Europe, bringing Christianity to Western Germany. In the year 800, Pope Leo III crowned him first king of the Holy Roman Empire.

This bit of history connects my grandfather's birthplace and my roots to a huge change in history. Gaul was made up of Celtic peoples whose Indo-European ancestors had migrated westward between 900 and 1200 B.C. Those who settled west of the Rhine became known as Celtic, while those east of the Rhine were Germanic. So, at one time, most of the people in Western Europe west of the Rhine were Celtic. It is they who conquered Great Britain. Presently, Celtic people with their related family of languages live in western France, Brittany, the Isle of Man, southeast England, Cornwall, Ireland, Wales, and Scotland.

Anatolians were a branch of Indo-European peoples who coexisted with populations from the north (Aryian-Persian) and east (Indian) about 7000 B.C. These Indo-Europeans spoke ancient languages such as those mentioned in Acts 2:9. Luke records at Pentecost people speaking in Parthians, Medes, Elamites and tongues from Mesopotamia. The trunk of the language tree branched first to the Anatolian language, then to Greek, Indian (Sanskrit), Iranian (Persian languages), Slovakian, Germanic, Romantic, and Armenian. Modern languages stemming from Indo-European languages include Bengali, English, French, Italian, Spanish, German, Russian, and Slovakian. The languages of about half the world's population have their roots in Indo-European languages. The Anatolian language tree disappeared with development of modern languages and no longer exists, but the central portion of Turkey is still called Anatolia. I have been interested in this phase of history because of the type of dogs I own and have raised and trained since 1969. The Brittany, or Epagneul Breton, as known in France, first came from Bretagne to the United States in the early 1930s. They possess traits of both spaniels and pointers.

Driving at 14

I learned to drive Grandpa Schaller's two-door, 1938 Chevrolet sedan on the gravel roads near the farm. Grandpa, being a bit crippled, was pleased to let me drive. Grandma, Grandpa, and I drove to Minot, North Dakota, where my mother's oldest sister, Florence, lived. The Boy With the Wounded Thumb drove most of the way except when coming to large towns, when we would stop and Grandpa Schaller would take over. After we had passed through a town, he stopped the car at the side of the road, and I resumed driving.

In Minot, we had a wonderful visit with Aunt Florence, who spoiled me from an early age. One day, Aunt Florence said, "Ma and Pa and Gordon, would you like to have dinner at a famous restaurant that serves buffalo steaks?"

I replied, "Yes, of course!"

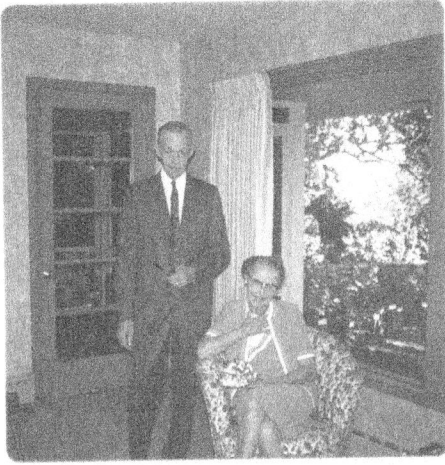

Aunt Florence and Don Zumbrook at home in Red Wing, Minnesota, 1960.

Florence made reservations in a nice hotel in downtown Minot. It was the first time I had stayed in a hotel – wow, what an experience. Shower, bathtub, huge towels, three times larger than I had ever seen before, and an evenly flat mattress on the bed. Florence introduced us to her friend, Don Zumbrook, who was an auto-parts salesman. Some years later they married and opened an auto-parts store in Red Wing, Minnesota. It was there, years later, that I saw the Redwing Boot Factory, and I own boots that were made there.

The journey continued from Minot to Greenbush, Minnesota, driving along highways just south of Canada. In Greenbush we stayed with Great Uncle Emile and Great Aunt Katie Schaller. They had four children: Clayton, Raymond, Anna Belle, and Florence. Grandpa had purchased a single-shot, 22-gauge rifle for me. I shot at crows in a grain field at great distance, but none were killed. Mosquitoes swarmed by the millions. Repellents were unavailable, so the flying, biting, blood-sucking insects had the upper hand.

Water-witching while visiting family

A trip to one of the largest lakes in Northern Minnesota, Lake of the Woods, about 20 miles east of Greenbush on the U.S.-Canada border, gave me the experience of discovering, for the first time in my life, a person with unusual special talent. A Sunday outing took us and several Emile Schaller family members by boat into Canadian territory. This was my first time in another country, and it was an exciting experience even though I never touched land. Travels to foreign countries would come starting 20 years later and bring opportunity to live a year in England and another year in Germany, as I'll describe in detail in *One Medicine War on Cancer.*

While at the Lake of the Woods picnic-park area, we were introduced to a "water witch." He was a "little person," and had the power to find underground water with a willow branch. I held the branch and walked along with him. Without him moving his hands, the willow would bend. My relatives told me that local farmers called upon him to find water underground to identify places for drilling wells. This same technique was used at our vacation home north of Gualala on the California Mendocino coast in 1970s. Many individuals have various types of special talents. Water witching, dowsing for underground water, is one special talent.

Fireflies

From Greenbush, we traveled south, staying overnight at a motel in Detroit Lakes, where I had another "first" experience. This time, it was exposure to fireflies. These insects fascinated me, and I remember them decades later. They are zoologically classified in the family *Lampyridae* and the beetle order of *Coleoptera*, winged beetles or lightning bugs. They have crepuscular (twilight) use of bioluminescence to attract mates or prey. This is an interesting way to attract a sex partner and a devious way to capture prey.

Fireflies' spectrum of cold light does not include infrared or ultraviolet frequencies; they produce light-wave frequencies in the range of 510 to 670 nanometers with color ranging from yellow and green to pale red. Fireflies have a light organ in the abdomen that is remarkably efficient in producing light without loss of energy through heat. The bioluminescence is produced by a chemical reaction within its body. The light-emitting organ contains calcium adenosine triphosphate (ATP), the substrate luciferin and the enzyme luciferase. The presence of oxygen triggers the reaction between these elements, resulting in light energy referred to as cold light. Many species have larva that glow, commonly known as glowworms.

Sometime after returning from our North Dakota-northern Minnesota trip, we traveled to Tracy in southwestern Minnesota, and visited with Uncle Charlie, my mother's oldest brother. Uncle Charlie was a fine man. He loved his wife, Audrey, and daughters, Ila May and Shirley. Charlie was farming land that seemed not too productive during financially difficult times. He gave off the body language of an unhappy man, yet was warm and wonderful to me. He was a special person whose personality was similar to that of his mother, my Grandma Schaller.

However, as it turns out, Audrey would step out with other men, leaving Charlie to care for the girls. In April of 1945, Charlie became seriously ill and died within two days from meningitis. Mom and Dad received a telegram from Grandma and Grandpa Schaller relating the news, which came as a huge shock. My parents were close to Uncle Charlie and immediately made arrangements to go by train to the funeral. I, at 16, was left in charge of the Richmond house and the responsibility of caring for my sister, Blythe. We two kids fared well in our parents' absence.

Return home via the Empire Builder: Flashback in time

I returned to Le Mars, Iowa, in August 1942 by the slow train from Maynard to Merrill. Two weeks later, I left for the West Coast on the Great Northern Railroad's Empire Builder train, which I boarded in Omaha, Nebraska, bound for Seattle. The trip brought back memories of cold winter days and nights on the Schields' farm, which was just a mile east of the tracks. The Great Northern engineer would toot the train whistle every day when the Empire Builder passed near our farm about 5 p.m.

I remembered one day, in the winter darkness of 1937, when it was as cold as it could be. Dad was chopping wood that I carried into the house for the pot-bellied stove when we heard the train whistle. Dad remarked, "Gordon, in three days that train will be in Seattle, and it will be warmer there." I never forgot that quip, and from that moment on I wanted to live someplace where it was much warmer than Minnesota in winter. This desire was not as strong as wanting to become a veterinarian like Dr. Rassmussen, but certainly the desire to be warm was strong.

Five years later there I was, traveling by myself on the Empire Builder to Seattle. The trip across the northern United States was fascinating, going through areas where Lewis and Clark had traveled some 165 years earlier and where my dad had traveled in his Model T Ford touring car some 20 years before. The train route went across northern North Dakota and northern Montana, and through Spokane, Washington, before ending at Seattle.

Aunt Louise, Uncle Ben's wife, met me at the station in Seattle. Ben was my Dad's older brother and was a very tall, standing six feet eight inches, just like my grandfather Henry Theilen. Ben and Louise lived in the Green Lake district of Seattle, a nice area that our family had visited in 1941. I had a good time in Seattle. Louise took me downtown to a coin shop and purchased an old U.S. coin for my collection. I had become interested in numismatics when collecting for my newspaper route. I would often get paid in small change, and started a penny, nickel, and dime collection that I discontinued after enlistment in the Army in 1946. I found one rare penny, a 1909 Lincoln minted in San Francisco with initials "VDB" on the back (honoring the coin's designer, Victor David Brenner). This is a very rare Lincoln head penny.

From Seattle, the Boy With the Wounded Thumb traveled south on the Western Pacific Railroad, and arrived home in Richmond in late August 1942. At the age of 14, I had traversed the country by train and car, covering some 6,000 miles on a trip inspired by dreaming about adventure in new places and the opportunity to visit relatives. I have always loved family ties and never stopped learning about my roots and places to visit.

I commenced junior high school as a ninth grader the first of September 1942. School remained on a half-day schedule because of overcrowding from the families of people who were pouring in to work at the shipyard and other defense factories that were springing up in the San Francisco Bay Area. Richmond was changing as it grew from a very friendly small East Bay town into a city with residents who had come from all parts of the nation, but mainly the Dust Bowl region and poor Southern states.

CHAPTER 12

Richmond High School, 1943–1946

Wisdom begins with reverence to God.
— Psalm 111:10

I made the transition in 1943 from ninth grade at Longfellow Junior High on 23rd Street, just south of MacDonald Avenue, to 10th grade at Richmond Union High School on 23rd about one mile north. This marked a big change in my developmental years, when I began to really enjoy educational experiences. Tenth grade was the beginning of my preparation for university and life as a responsible citizen equipped to work in various vocations or to join the military. Many high school students enlisted in military service after graduation, while others went directly to higher education or began a full-time job.

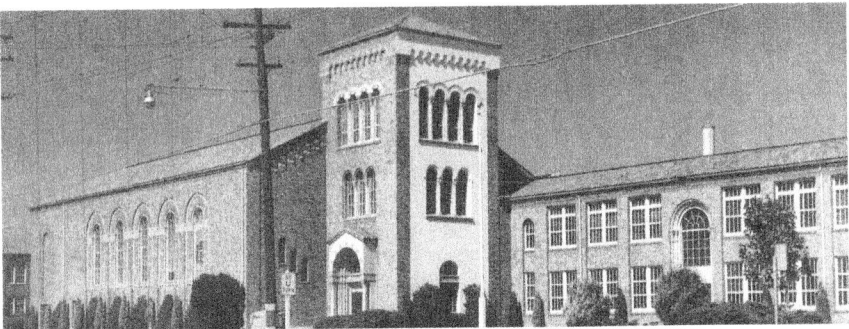

Richmond Union High School.

The main high school building was on two levels, with broad access ramps at both ends. It was an impressive structure made of red brick. The wide front entrance was set off by a granite boulder four feet high engraved "Richmond Union High School." Behind the building were a metal shop, wood shop, and a maintenance building for school buses. The athletic fields included a football stadium with a track and a baseball diamond. The school also had a gym where basketball and other indoor sports were played. The Richmond School District included the towns of San Pablo, El Sobrante, Hercules, and Pinole. It extended on Highway 4 to the Martinez School District border, and north as far as Rodeo. Students were bused from the outer reaches of the district.

Leonard Morhing: Lifetime of coincidences

A class member, Leonard Morhing, lived on a ranch near Highway 4 and the southern border of the Martinez School district. The Morhing family's ranch bordered the Pereira family's ranch to the south. The school district lines ran between ranches, and the Pereira kids went to Martinez High School. After I retired from UC Davis in 1993, I discovered that a former Martinez student, Henry Pereira, lived across the road from our retirement home in Dixon. This was one of many interesting coincidences in my life as my classmate Leonard Morhing and Henry Pereira were good neighborly friends while in high school, yet went to different schools because of school district boundaries.

Subject disciplines and teachers

In the tenth grade I took algebra, French I, English, Chemistry I, and other classes. I was intimidated by French and barely passed the course. Blanche Carson, the French instructor, took our class to San Francisco to dine at an authentic French restaurant whose walls were plastered with posters of the Eiffel Tower, Notre Dame, a bridge across the Seine, and other French landmarks. This was a marvelous experience and the first time I had exposure to a five-course meal. First, we cleansed our palates with sorbet, then supped delicious onion soup, salad, and a meat course with yummy white sauce covered with mushrooms. All the while we were eating French bread. The meal finished with a light pastry.

Blanche had spent time in France before the war and had an inspiring method of teaching. I took French again in the eleventh grade to obtain credit for the two years of foreign language needed to qualify for entrance to the University of California. Little did I know that 20 years later, on a job-related trip to France, I would make good use of that high school French.

My experience in France was that French citizens on the street in Paris and other large cities ignored foreigners who asked questions in English. They would reply if I initially spoke in French, and would continue speaking to me even after I switched to English. I found people in the rural areas more hospitable and helpful in assisting with directions and finding hotels and restaurants, and generally they were more open to speaking with a foreign visitor.

Carolyn and I traveled extensively by car in France in 1979 and 1980 and were able to communicate nicely using high-school French. I will cherish exposure to my first foreign language in Blanche Carson's class. I remember and revere her as an educator, a superb teacher full of enthusiasm. Her influence was enormous and led me to a lifetime of enthusiastic teaching at UC Davis.

With opportunity to travel extensively over the years as a cancer researcher, I was exposed to many languages and along the way learned a bit of Japanese, Indonesian, Danish, Dutch, Norwegian, Swedish, and German, and I improved my French. German became a second language for Carolyn and me; we lived in Germany for a year, and we retain much of it 30 years later.

Another class of special note was Mr. France's public speaking class. I had a public speaking fear, and intuition led me to enroll in his class. His instruction indeed got me over my fear, and what I learned was useful when I became a faculty member at UC Davis. The main technique was to look straight at the audience and imagine all were naked. Wow, this helped overcome a huge barrier!

Mr. France was the only teacher from my high school who wrote a note in my January 1945 yearbook. "Gordon, I would hardly say that it was always inspiration to learn that all your actions in class were well attended; but believe it or not I've enjoyed your presence in my class. Signed, Robert France."

James Ice taught my sophomore chemistry IA course in 1944, and Arthur Sellick taught my chemistry IB course. These classes were extremely interesting, and I gained knowledge that put me ahead of others in Chem IA/IB at the University of California, Berkeley, in 1949. In high school we had partners to share needed supplies for various chemical experiments. My partner was Delores Stroski, who married classmate Ted Abbott in June 1946.

Mr. Sellick, our IA/IB physics instructor, had a Ph.D. degree. He was a serious man who seemed out of touch with everyday happenings despite a higher learning degree. For instance, on one occasion he asked classmate Ken Wells a question. Ken was silent for a time, and then Mr. Sellick said, "Ken, speak up!" Ken replied, "awruff, awruff," which had the class roaring with laughter. The class was a bit rowdy and would hide things from Mr. Sellick before he arrived at 1 p.m. to unlock the classroom door. He was always late because he taught a class from noon to 1. He locked the classroom door so we could not get in until he arrived. On warm fall days, the first-floor windows were left open because the school had no air conditioning. Sometimes the temperature would get close to 100 degrees F. Some of my classmates crawled through the open windows and placed gum in the door's keyhole. Mr. Sellick could not get in, although his students were all present. These were among the pranks we played on teachers while in high school.

Grace Condon was our typing instructor. Through her, I learned typing technique that has carried me through to the computer age. Robert Sikes taught civics, and his lessons have come into play many times with regard to our Constitution and its use in our government. It was a well-taught class. F.L Culbertson taught fundamentals of mechanical drawing, which also came in handy on many occasions after high school.

Phil Hempler taught physical education, which emphasized attainment of physical fitness through various types of sports. He was the track coach, and during our years at Richmond High the track team excelled. Especially outstanding were the 220 and 440 relay teams made up of Dwayne McClendon, Larry Hoff, Richard Kaufman, and Bob Kershaw. Hoff was an excellent 110 and 220 hurdler. Ralph Daniel was a good 440 and half-mile runner. Mr. Hempler had been a track star at the UC Berkeley in the 1930s. He attended our 50th class reunion. At the time he was in his 90s, but he still flashed the friendly smile that I remember when he was teaching at Richmond High School.

Mr. Hempler kept the baton that the 1945 rely track team used in winning the Divisional Championship. After his death, his son gave the bamboo baton to Ron Kamb, a classmate, and somehow the baton miraculously was given to Rich Kaufman, the anchor man on the team, at the Richmond High School alumni breakfast on August 13, 2015. The baton from this famous high school relay team had been passed back to a classmate and track team member 69 years later, a coincidence of massive proportions.

Helen Hoefer was my algebra and geometry teacher. When she handed me the algebra book for course use on first day of the 1943 fall term, she said, "Gordon I hope you are a better student than he who had this book 16 years ago." See, it was used by a kid who was left-handed, and his nickname was Lefty. He was a good pitcher for the Richmond High baseball team, then went from playing with the San Francisco Seals to become a starting pitcher for the New York Yankees, known to fans as Lefty Gomez. Wow, a famous baseball pitcher learned algebra from the same book I was using! That increased my zeal for baseball, and I have become an avid San Francisco Giants baseball fan. I rally enjoyed algebra and was good overall in mathematics, but I found geometry, which I studied in the 1944 fall term, challenging.

Alice Vorheis taught advanced English. Her class was devoted to ancient and modern literature. We discussed and studied ancient writings by Plato and Socrates. We read and studied Chaucer and several plays by Shakespeare, parts of which we re-enacted. This class left a lifelong impression of the beauty and mind-broadening thinking that characterizes good literature. I frequently read books written by deep-thinking authors, and the Holy Bible, which was not discussed in Mrs. Vorheis's classroom despite the fact that many of Shakespeare's quotes came directly from Holy Scripture. As years went on, I developed an insatiable passion about various types of writing. However, I never developed appreciation for poetry.

I frequently quote Shakespeare. I recall doing so to good effect on one occasion when I was traveling with my dogs and good friend, Rick Green, to participate in a field trial at the California City area of the Mohave Desert. The day before, one of my dogs while eating kibble spilled feed on the gravel ground and ingested a fairly large pebble. She became ill with an intestinal blockage on a cold, windy January night. By early morning, the pebble had moved to the colon and near the rectum, and it was obvious it would pass. I quoted Shakespeare: "She was plucked from a dense nettle forest and brought to safety." I frequently quote Winston Churchill, an exceptionally well read and versed man. My favorite recalled Churchill expression is, "On such small points of agates does the world revolve." Mrs. Vorheis's lessons in good literature opened pathways for future experiences and an enjoyable life.

Ms. Bryns, a UC Berkeley graduate, was the Subject A English teacher. She was furious with an essay I had written and gave an "F." She asked where I intended to attend college. When I answered, "UC Berkeley," she immediately replied, "Don't bother, *you won't make it."* I ended the course with a "D," which meant I had to take "bonehead English" when I entered UC Berkeley. Ms. Bryns had suggested that the Boy With the Wounded Thumb was too much of a bonehead to succeed at UC Berkeley. She did not know that I wanted to become a veterinarian since I was 5 years old and had never wavered. This incident turned out to be a blessing in disguise. From the day I began teaching at UC Davis until the day I retired, I never in 37 and a half years, no matter how displeased I was with a student, said *"you will never make it."*

On the gridiron

Neal Wade was the coach of the Richmond High School football team, the Oilers. I played on the junior varsity team but remember little of the 1943 season. The team of 1944–45 included linemen Ken Wells, Bill Sproule, Dick Macfie, Blair Smith, Bob Wier, Ernie Liebhardt, and Al Robertson. The backfield consisted of Ed Bond, Leroy McGrue, Rich Kaufman, and Everett Babb, with me at quarterback. The second-string team was made up of other good players, in particular Ray Moitosa and Al Harris. I developed lifelong friendships with several teammates. Some friendships that had begun when I was in sixth grade and continued at Longfellow Junior High flourished in high school and have endured beyond. Mr. Wade taught discipline, desire to succeed, the importance of being a strong member of the team, and the value of working together. Those were lessons I applied in my professional career, as I realized that success in research depended on creating a research team, a "critical mass," to make new discoveries.

Our 1945 season was not one to cheer about, but wasn't bad either.

Richmond	Opponent	
33	Napa	0
19	San Rafael	12
6	Alameda	12
7	Albany	13
0	Piedmont	13
6	El Cerrito	6

| 25 | St. Mary's | 8 |
| 7 | Berkeley | 32 |

The game against Hayward was forfeited.

It took hard physical work and practice to condition for football. One game I fondly remember was against El Cerrito at our stadium. We battled back and forth for a good three quarters in a no-score game. Then El Cerrito scored and did not make the conversion. Al Robertson and I had practiced long passes, and in the fourth quarter, I called a long pass-play from our 20-yard line. I faked a handoff to Rich Kaufman, coming through as if attempting to gain yardage on the ground; then ran backward about 10 yards turned around with the ball as the opposing team reacted to tackle Kaufman, and I threw a long pass of perhaps 40 yards to Al. He was a fast runner, caught it going away, and ran for a tie-scoring touchdown. We missed the point after, and the rest of the game was back-and-forth that ended in a tie. We were happy just to tie what we thought was a better team, as their record indicated.

My relationship with Dick Macfie was special. We played on the sixth-grade touch-football team and continued a close association throughout high school. He was a good student and acknowledged as the most outstanding scholar on the fall 1945 football squad. We later belonged to the same fraternity, Sigma Chi, at UC Berkeley. I was honored to serve as best man for the wedding of Dick and Lil (née Sernack).

We saw little of each other after I transferred from UC Berkeley to UC Davis in 1950, but we again saw each other frequently when I was doing a fellowship at the National Cancer Institute (NCI). Dick was assigned to the Office of the Chief of Naval Operations at the Pentagon in Alexandria, Virginia. Unfortunately, he and his son, Andy, were in a nasty car ancient. Dick was taken to the National Naval Medical Center at Bethesda, Maryland, across Wisconsin Avenue from NCI at the National Institutes of Health campus. Even though it was a considerable distance from NCI, I could easily see the National Naval Medical Center's white 15-story tower from there.

Andy suffered severe head trauma in that accident, and was in intensive care for several weeks. He needed a series of brain surgeries. The night of the accident, Lil, Carolyn, and I knelt at the hospital chapel chancel railing and prayed for Andy and Dick's survival and recovery. Andy's life was in the balance for several days, but he has survived into his 50s. Dick was hospitalized for three months. Through the years we have remained the best of friends. I have been blessed with friendships, in my childhood, in high school and college, through Christian affiliations, academic colleagues, veterinary clients, dog owners, and friends from all walks of life.

Other happenings

As a result of losing a bet with Larry Hoff, a fellow track team member, Rich Kaufman was to run the high school corridors in a jockstrap. He was a fast runner, but this was the run of his life. Mrs. Phillips came out of her classroom just in time to see him. She screeched and yelled out, "What are you doing? You are obscene, something has to be done about this!"

She immediately went to the principal's office, demanding Rich's expulsion. Principal Gray summoned Rich, and after Rich explained what happened and pled for leniency, Mr. Gray said he thought the whole affair was hilarious. He had never seen Mrs. Phillips so upset. She had been a thorn in his side, and he suggested that Rich's prank was not a big deal.

In the spring of 1946, Dick Macfie and Dwayne McClendon were sailing off Point Richmond in Dick's small sailboat. Waves capsized them late in the afternoon, and Dick and Dwayne swam to a nearby rocky island, where they were marooned all night. They were rescued the next morning in a state of hypothermia. Some time later, classmates Dick Mythen and Marshall Smith drowned when their small sailboat capsized in the same area.

Beginning sixty-five years after graduation, several members of the class began meeting monthly for get-together breakfasts. Ten of us gathered in 2010 at Lake Forest Café in Folsom, California.

In the summer of 1944, I attended High Y camp at Garberville, on the Russian River. We had play and swim time when free learning about Hi Y earning achievement scarves. Ron Nicholson's younger brother drowned, leaving the boys in camp shocked. A week or so later, Ron and I closed up camp and drove in Ron's Model A pickup from Garberville to Richmond. The only way to go directly to Richmond was to take the Richmond-San Rafael ferry. The last boat left at 11:30 p.m., and we missed it. This meant we had to drive a roundabout route across the Golden Gate Bridge, through San Francisco, across the Bay Bridge, then north along the East Bay to Richmond. We arrived at 4 a.m., causing our parents much anxiety in the process.

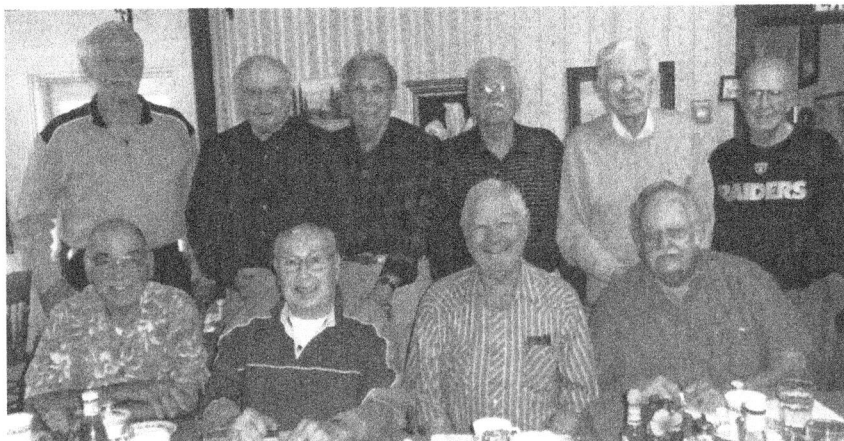

Ten Richmond high school graduates at Lake Forest Café in 2010. Standing (left to right) were Ken Wells, Ron Kamb, John Howard, Rich Kaufman, Ralph Daniel, Clyde Ferria; seated left to right were Sharf Hazarbidian, Ray Mantoza, Gordon Theilen, and Bob Feenan.

Jolly Boys

A group of six boys – Dick Macfie, Dick McGranahan, Rich Kaufman, Dwayne McClendon, Ernie Liebhardt and I – loosely had a self-organized fraternity called the Jolly Boys. We got together Friday nights and dined in Chinese restaurants at Chinatown in San Francisco. Chopsticks were required. One evening, we decided that by the following week, each of us would have a steady girlfriend. Up to our senior year, none of us had a steady girlfriend. By that next week, we all were committed to dating only one girl. I asked Jerry Scales, and she and I continued to go steady until I entered the U.S. Army in September 1946.

On my 18th birthday, Mom prepared a surprise dinner party. When I came home, the Jolly Boys were all sitting at the table. Mom made a wonderful meal and baked an angel food cake, one of my favorites. Some of the Jolly Boys still remember and talk about that meal. Three of us – Ernie Leibhardt, Rich Kaufman and I – continued seeing each other frequently well into adulthood, until Ernie died. They recalled my Mom as a person who had concerns about my friends and helped them in numerous ways. Mom and Dad always had the door open for my friends, and the many meals Mom prepared were scrumptious. Ours was a happy, friendly home.

High school years were special and planted seeds of enthusiasm in the hearts and minds of many of us who graduated in the mid 1940s. It prepared us for living productive lives with contributions to our families. The marriages of very few of us ended in separations, as our generation was pro-marriage, pro-life, not involved in the drug culture, and overall committed to a Judeo-Christian moral ethic. The Boy With the Wounded Thumb was educated and lived in the Golden Era of the American Dream.

Teenage years

High-school days spanned late childhood and into puberty. These transition years meant male and female friends took on different relationships. The subtleness of these early relationships gave urges to find the special girl; in my case it took many dates. The first girl I kissed was at a teenage party held by Ralph Pinchon's mom at their home. Before, parties I'd attended were gatherings of only boys. We would play cards and tell stories. At this party, girls and boys played various games, one of which was spin the bottle. We sat in a circle and took turns spinning the bottle in the middle of the circle. When the bottle stopped, the spinner would kiss the girl at whom the neck of the bottle pointed. I had my first kiss that way, and the girl was Jane Thornton. Sometime in my junior year, I asked her out to a weekend Hi-Y dance. When I saw her to the door after the dance, I said goodnight without offering a kiss.

Jane was a student at the Anna Head School for Girls, a private high school in Berkeley, and we would frequently see each other at teenage doings in Richmond. She was present at times at high school functions and wrote a note in my fall and spring issues of the Richmond High School Shield Yearbooks – "Lots of luck, be seeing ya, Jane Thornton." The next time I saw Jane was fall of 1948 on the UC Berkeley campus, where she was a coed. We had a nice chat. Many years later, at breakfast with high school classmates Ron Cole and others, I learned that Jane was on the board of directors of Mechanics Bank. The bank, which her grandfather had founded in San Pablo, California, had expanded and grown to several branches of substantial monetary wealth. Jane developed breast cancer, and a short time after I learned about her malady in 2009, she died.

I will always remember that first kiss, not because of being in love, but because special, warm relationships develop when close contact of closed lips becomes a landmark event in the process of becoming a man.

Quotes from *Blue Shield* yearbooks

JUNE 1944 YEARBOOK: The signature of Ralph Pinchon recalls a good friend and most sincere person I ever met. "To a swell guy," wrote Pat Sutton. "Best wishes always, to a swell fella," Barbara Schulze wrote.

JANUARY 1945 EDITION: "To a fellow ravioli eater" – Marshall Smith. (Marshall drowned in a boating accident sometime after graduation.) "To a swell pal since Longfellow. Lots of luck always" – Pat Sutton. "Study a little harder next term and maybe you'll get that big A in Chem" – Dolores Straski. "To a swell fellow and wonderful dancer" – Alice Bench. One signature was that of "Don Cheeks Sagner." Don had reddish cheeks and was frequently reminded about his rosiness. Don is a member of the Richmond High breakfast group that meets once a month. "To a blond diago and spaghetti eater, lots of luck" – Joe Felise. Friends in high school had different skin colors or religious preferences, but I did not regard certain colors of skin or religious preferences as requirements to be a friend.

"To a pal" wrote Everett Babb," a fellow football player who remained a good friend. "Lots of luck," wrote Gerrie Scales. A year and some months later, Gerrie became a steady girlfriend of mine. She was special and a nice young person. "Good luck to a fellow football pal," Ken Wells wrote. Ken remained a friend.

"To the moron with the Highest I.Q. in school" – Mildred Wiegers. Others referred to me as a student with imagination and intellect, yet I was far from being an A student. I preferred absorbing substance material rather than details for a test.

"To a swell person, also a very humorous one with Mr. France," Marie Sartori wrote. Mr. France taught good lessons for public speaking. When first exposed to public speaking, even in a classroom setting, I was speechless. "To one of the nicest, friendliest guys I know. Best wishes, Dolores Whiteman." She was a speech classmate.

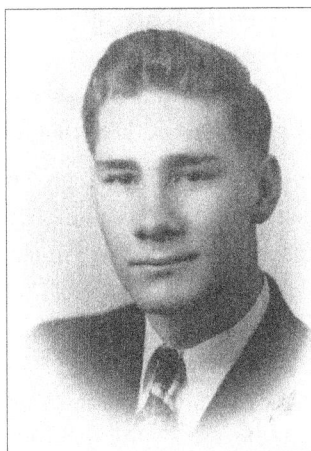

My high school graduation photo.

91

JUNE 1945 SHIELD: That issue included quotes from many others. "Here's to a darn swell fellow, and one of the Tri Y, Sierra Club, Loads of luck," Bill Pedrick wrote. Bill became an army cadet at West Point right after graduation. In 1946, he and fellow classmate George Manning were flying home for Christmas on a military plane that crashed, killing all on board. This tragedy was deeply felt in the Richmond community because they were known young men from respected families. Suddenly, everyone was in mourning.

"The best always to a wonderful football player, and a sweet fellow, and a wonderful friend. May that friendship last as it has in the past. – Lorraine Johnson. P.S. Pretty good snow pictures you take." Lorraine was a girlfriend I often dated but with whom I had frequent disagreements. She became the steady girlfriend of Bob Costello, who was a fellow football player and in 1939 lived near us on 18th Street near Gaynor. Bob was bigger at that time and a bit older, giving him the advantage in a fistfight with me that he won. Needless to say, he was not one of my best friends for several reasons. Some years later, after graduation, he and Lorraine married. I saw them at our 25th class reunion. Shortly after, Bob died. I never saw Lorraine again. She, too, was a nice and outstanding young lady.

"Dear Gordon, Je vous aime, Je vous adore. Que vouley-vous Je fais encore? Votre amie," written in 1945. Nancie Fallman wrote. In the February 1946 yearbook, Nancie wrote "To dear, conceited Gordon, no kiddin', you're a wonderful guy 'n I loves ya." The quote in French is more than amorous, and perhaps I was not as observant about Nancie's friendship as I should have been. Had I understood French better, I might have gotten a clear message. I was not a good French student, which left me out on a friendship limb.

"Theilen, my friend," Leroy McGrue wrote. He was football teammate and a sincere friend who in the February edition of the Shield wrote, "To a pal who played some fine ball, but didn't get much credit for it. I will remember you for the rest of my life. Wish we were playing another year. – Leroy McGrue '46." Leroy was one of the commencement speakers at our graduation. He became a Christian minister in Vallejo as a member of the black community and was pastor of a black congregation. He was recognized in Vallejo, where a street was named in his memory. Unfortunately, I never saw Leroy after the 25th class reunion that was held in Vallejo.

"2/6/46, dear Gordie. The best of everything to you always, You really deserve it. You have personality, looks, and brains. Nuff said here," Barbara Schulze wrote. "To a swell guy and a good Hi member. Remember the El Cerrito game when we were in our glory? – Al (El Cerrito) Robertson." Al died at a very early age from a heart attack. The Boy With the Wounded Thumb remembers the El Cerrito game better than any other games played in high school.

I remember a severe right ankle sprain in the game against Napa in the fall of 1943. When I was performing a quarterback sneak, a player fell on the back of my leg. The ankle swelled like a balloon, and in those days, the doctor was Mom. The treatment consisted of hot compresses soaked in Epsom salts (magnesium sulfate) and Ace bandaging for several days, followed by a limping walk for several weeks.

There were many more quotes from various yearbooks. Those I remember best are from members of the breakfast group that meets once a month. Twenty-five years after graduation, Dick Macfie told me, "Gordie, you were the only one in our class that stuck by what you wanted to be."

High school dances

School dances were well chaperoned and sanctioned by the Hi-Y branch of the YMCA and Tri-Y equivalent at the YWCA. Between their events and high school dances or prom, there was opportunity to dance every weekend. Local bands would play for special events, but usually we danced to recordings of famous dance bands of the 1940s. The music of Benny Goodman, Tommy Dorsey, Glenn Miller, and others bring back memories to those days.

In the tenth and eleventh grades, I dated several girls. At dances, it was customary to dance the first and last dance with one's date and the rest of the dances with girls other boys had brought. Gerrie Scales, Lillian Cox, Patricia Donogh, Pat Waldon, Molly Hokanson, Rosemary Milicevich, Carol Claar, Joyce Evenson, Loraine Johnson, Miriam Tillman, Peggy Humphrey, Barbara Schulze, Jane Thornton, Janice Nelson, Dorris Sullivan, Lucille Mallan, Nona Kaufman, Nancie Fallman, Betty Iman, June Smith, and Dolores Whiteman were among the girls I dated. I stayed in touch through the years with Barbara Schulze, whose memorial service I attended in 2010; and Lucille Mallan, who came to my 80th birthday celebration in May 2009. The Sierra Hi-Y met once a week, and after the meeting, the group would go to various girls' homes for refreshments and chatter with one another. At Lucille Mallan's home she would always play "Stairway to the Stars" on the piano. I have such fond memories of the days of 1944 to 1946. Our togetherness as students spanned a total of no more than three years, yet some remain glued together 70 and more years.

Summer vacation work

I worked in the summers of 1945 and 1946 at the Standard Oil refinery in Richmond. The refinery, at Point Richmond, inspired our high-school football team's name, the Oilers. Standard oil hired teenagers to work at the refinery, as a large proportion of the adult work force was in military service. In my first summer there I worked in the asphalt still, where 50-gallon drums filled with flowing asphalt liquid at 250 degrees Fahrenheit came down a conveyor, from which they were placed on pallets wide enough for six barrels. I was taught to roll the 550-pound barrels onto the pallets, using my thighs to balance the heavy barrels. A jitney would take the pallets to a cooling area before loading them onto railway cars headed for wherever asphalt was needed to build military landing strips on islands in the Pacific Theater of World War II. This was heavy labor, and my first few days of learning to roll the heavy barrels filled with searing hot asphalt resulted in first- and second-degree burns on my thighs. My mother sewed pads on the thigh portions of my blue jeans for protection. Any liquid asphalt spilled on the floor had to be cleaned immediately; if permitted to harden, it had to be chipped free.

Exposure to veterinary medicine

Dr. Seymour Roberts **was** a general veterinary practitioner in Richmond whose practice hospital was on the west side of San Pablo Avenue north of Barrett Avenue. I told him I was interested in veterinary medicine and wondered if he had a job available. He told me that he needed kennels cleaned and janitorial work done in late afternoons. I worked for him from 1944 to 1946 after school and on weekends.

Dr. Roberts had received his DVM degree from Michigan State University College of Veterinary Medicine. Parts of Richmond were semirural when he began his practice there as a general practitioner, so he took large-animal calls and performed tasks on small farms with a milking cow or two, a few sheep or goats, a horse, pigs, and poultry. I assisted in castrating a two-year-old stallion. Castration was done with no anesthetic. The horse was restrained using ropes and hobbles and was tripped. The legs were tied above the hoofs to keep the animal on his back and prevent him from rising. After the castration, the ropes were removed and the animal was allowed to get up with a bit of blood dripping between his legs. The wound was not sutured, and he was given only a vaccine to prevent tetanus.

I also participated in removing a retained placenta from a cow after it gave birth. I did many retained placenta procedures in my career, by inserting my arm into the cow's vagina and gently removing the attached placenta. If not removed, the placenta can be retained for several days. With no blood supply, the tissue becomes infected and turns a dark brownish hue, with a strong smell of deteriorating bacterial contaminated dead tissue.

Dr. Roberts was pleased with my assistance and soon asked me to help in small-animal surgeries. I served as his anesthetist when the assistant was not available. It was an exciting exposure to veterinary medicine. I saw surgeries, usually neutering of dogs and cats. I was introduced to ether and chloroform anesthetics administered by aerosol inhalation, using a small cone containing cotton soaked in the anesthetic. A small margin of error was in play, as excessive anesthetic would lead to cessation of heart and breathing functions. Frequently, Dr. Roberts would say, "Back off on the cone until the animal starts to breathe again." Chloroform had a sweet odor, while ether had a distinct and unique medicinal odor. In the 1980s and 1990s, anesthesiology became more exacting science with injectable and inhaled anesthetics that decreased surgical procedure mortality.

Dr. Roberts increased my weekend responsibilities to include administering of medications, orally and eventually by subcutaneous or intramuscular injections. He eventually gave me total responsibility in administering medications and recording overall health and bodily functions on the daily health chart. With the guidance of Dr. Roberts, I had developed into a capable animal technician by the time I graduated from high school. Animal technicians with special training became a recognized sub-specialty of veterinary medicine two to three decades later.

I learned to "read" animals to determine if I needed assistance in holding the patient while giving medications, or if it could be done alone. Animals can be easily upset and resist medication, or can be assured that no harm will come to them. When hospitalized, an animal is in a strange and foreign environment, often for the first time.

Animals have fantastic memories and can forever remember unpleasant experiences, just as they will fondly remember loving care. I recall one dog as excessively aggressive. It was a red American cocker spaniel that would lunge and show its teeth when I approached the cage. The whites of the eyes (sclera) were bloodshot red. It was impossible for me to orally treat this dog. Yet a cleaning lady, unable to write or read, could take the dog out of the cage to an outside run while cleaning its cage. From this, I learned that fear shown by a human caring for an animal often brings on aggression. The cleaning lady could not read the sign on the cage, "Danger, do not touch the dog, it must be snared to move to an outside run," and thus she was not afraid. I was never bitten by a cat or dog in my care anytime during my veterinary career, because I was able to read them. This ability came from childhood exposure to animals and work with Dr. Roberts and later with Dr. Robert Walker in Pleasanton.

Veterinary ophthalmology practice

Dr. Roberts took a day off each week to go to Stanford Medical School, which was developing advanced science in human ophthalmology – eye medicine and surgery. He became the first practicing veterinarian in the United States to conduct a specialty of veterinary ophthalmology. Dr. Roberts advised me that when I became a veterinarian, I should do something special and unique that no one else has done in the profession. Little did he know that the Boy With the Wounded Thumb would become the first person in the world to develop the specialty of veterinary cancer medicine and would be the discoverer of the mammalian sarcoma virus, Snyder-Theilen feline sarcoma, the simian sarcoma virus and the reticuloendotheleosis virus from turkeys. I was able to ride on the shoulders of inspiring pioneers like Dr. Roberts who provided examples of ways to excel.

Dr. Roberts was a low-key person who was observant and interested in improving practice skills. Initially, I asked him if I could take time off Sunday mornings to go to church, which was about two miles away. Getting there by bicycle meant being away from the veterinary clinic for two hours, from 10:30 a.m. to 12:30 p.m. I always appreciated his granting this request. He was an excellent man in many ways and wrote a letter of recommendation for me. I'm sure his letter was helpful in my admission to veterinary school in 1951. I am grateful for that opportunity to work with a pioneering veterinarian, the first to practice ophthalmology. I was blessed to be first in several veterinary endeavors that helped animal owners by improving overall knowledge of comparative cancer problems. As a high-school student I had a veterinary mentor, an opportunity that most veterinary and Ph.D. students never experience, and working with Dr. Roberts was an important cornerstone in my career.

My graduation from Richmond High School on June 19, 1946, led to a starkly different phase of my life.

Richmond Union High School
Richmond, California

This Certifies that
Gordon Henry Theilen
has completed a course of studies in accordance with the requirements of the State Board of Education and the Trustees of this School and is therefore awarded this Diploma

Given at Richmond, California this fourteenth day of June, nineteen hundred and forty-six

President Board of Trustees

Superintendent of Schools

Principal

My high school graduation diploma, 1946.

CHAPTER 13

United States Army, 1946–1948

"I know, my dear Watson, that you share my love of all that is bizarre and outside the conventions and humdrum routine of everyday life."
– Sherlock Holmes

The summer of 1946 was a time of melancholy between high school graduation and enlistment in the U.S. Army. I had deep-seated thoughts of graduation from high school and the loss of my association with close friends. Three high school years brought enjoyment in learning and contentment in living. Before my life was always in throes of what I needed to do next to help my family make ends meet. I was, always in need until 1942. Concerns were obvious about coming mature commitments – entering adulthood and unknown challenges ahead to gain a degree in veterinary medicine. I was among thirty high-school classmates who enlisted in the Army at the same time in San Francisco, then were bused to Camp Beale, east of Marysville, on September 3. World War II had not yet come to a complete conclusion, with unrest persisting in Europe and areas of the Pacific. Communism was on the rise around the world; Zionists were planning to establish a new country in British-controlled Palestine.

Congress in 1944 had passed the Servicemen's Readjustment Act, commonly known as the G.I. Bill, which upon completion of service duty guaranteed financial assistance for "government issue" servicemen to attend college. Most classmates intended to go to college and did on the G.I. Bill, making considerable contributions to our country's educated work force. Military service would help fund my college education.

Camp Beale, Marysville, California

It was 98 degrees Fahrenheit in San Francisco and 112 degrees at Camp Beale on the day we were bussed. Upon arrival, we were assigned to a bunk in a barracks, given vaccination shots, and issued winter clothing – including woolen pants, shirts, and coats. We had to wear that, in 112-degree weather. Fatigue clothes were also issued. Long lines awaited in the hot, bright Sierra foothills sun. The ground was dry, with no trees for shade. This part of California normally has no rain from early summer to late fall. With little rain, summer is a time for dormancy, much as winter is a time of dormancy in colder climes.

Immunizations against infectious diseases were administered by medics with nurse assistants holding large forceps wrapped in cotton soaked with iodine to swab bare upper arms. Several recruits instantly became unsteady, turned pale and collapsed one after the other, almost like a fainting epidemic, all resulting from anticipation associated with vaccinations. The temporarily decreased blood supply to the brain was quickly reversed, and unconscious recruits were again on their feet. A few, however, remained unconscious or unsteady, probably from slight heat stroke or dehydration, and needed a stay in the infirmary to recover fully. Mass fainting episodes are psychologically initiated by heat, with fatigue acting as a contributing factor. This was the only time I saw a large number of persons fainting during the same procedure.

"Gray ladies" about the age of our mothers greeted us with kindness and hospitality, giving us free Camel cigarettes in six-packs. Most of the recruits had not been smokers before then. This free six-pack of cigarettes was the first for me, and led to a nicotine addiction lasting until my marriage to Carolyn in 1953. I quit smoking after our short honeymoon and never smoked again.

Also staying in our barracks were some soldiers who had returned from the battlefields of Europe and the Pacific. One was a heavily wounded paratrooper from the 503rd regiment of the 82nd Airborne Division who impressed me as he told about being in a hospital for several months as result of being wounded in Germany shortly before the Germans surrendered in May of 1945. His uniform was adorned with a large number of ribbons. A Purple Heart and Bronze Star for valor were proudly displayed on his chest. An aiguilette (ornamental braided cord) adorned each of his shoulders, with objects looking like miniature bells hanging at the ends. These aiguilettes were given by the French Army to the 82nd Airborne for heroism in helping to liberate France. They were an impressive reminder of the personal sacrifice made by our forces to keep America free from tyranny and terrorism.

A sergeant would come through the barracks and enlist recruits for KP (kitchen patrol) duty. I was recruited on the second day after arrival and was told the duty would be an eight-hour shift. The kitchen was fiercely hot, with no air conditioning. Most meats were fatty and cooked in large containers. A noticeable stench filled the air when grease was taken to the disposal drum outside the kitchen, covered with flies attracted to the rancid contents of the barrel. We peeled potatoes using a small knife, which resulted in a large amount of waste because recruits were not professional cooks. On KP, we frequently cleaned tables and mopped floors.

The mess hall was in continuous use. As new recruits arrived and stepped off the buses, they were first given food before assignments. After each meal, metal dinner trays were washed, placed in the dishwasher, and then stacked. It was go, go, go, hour after hour. Relief never came at the so-called end of my eight-hour shift. After KP for 16 hours with no relief, I returned to the barracks for rest. This was the first and only occasion during my 18 months in the military that I walked away from assigned duty.

Train ride to Fort Knox, Kentucky

Four days later, we set out on a train ride to Fort Knox, Kentucky, dressed in woolen clothes and carrying our green Army duffel bags, which substituted for suitcases during the remainder of our enlistment period. Daytime temperatures when we left Camp Beale were greater than 100 degrees F, and hot weather remained with us through the first several days of travel. The troop train was not air-conditioned, and the seats were uncomfortable. We opened windows to let air into the stuffy car.

The train moved from Marysville to the main track toward Southern California. We traveled through the Mojave Desert east to Flagstaff, Albuquerque, down to El Paso, crossed Texas and Louisiana into Mississippi, headed north through Tennessee, and on the fifth day arrived in Fort Knox. It was an indirect way, but probably routed specifically for troop train travel. Our troop train was sidetracked to wait as commercial trains passed. We went five days without showers, and the smell of body odor had become apparent after the first two. The olfactory mechanisms kicked in at first, but after a few days, the sense of smell became fatigued and all were oblivious, not only to body odor, but also to the fact that we looked more like ragamuffins than recently inducted Army recruits. The toilets became a mess and often were out of paper. This was the third train trip for the Boy With the Wounded Thumb but was not nearly as exciting as the prior train rides. However, it added to my experiences in seeing the vast country of the United States, from the deserts of the Southwest to the magnolia trees of the deep South, the greenness of the Ohio Valley Basin, and the rolling hills around Fort Knox, the place where the U.S. government stored vast quantities of gold and precious metals.

Basic training

We were assigned to basic artillery training for eight weeks without leave. The 18-year-old recruits just out of high school were no longer boys, but men being trained for fighting a war with 55-millimeter howitzer artillery. Every soldier was assigned an Army rifle not much different from a .30-06 caliber hunting rifle.

We did rigorous calisthenics, and everywhere we went, we marched in order. We wore our dress uniforms with all brass emblems highly polished. Our uniforms had shoulder patches identifying us as part of the artillery, and an emblem designating rank. All of us began as privates, with one strip on the left shoulder of the dress coat. Boots were rough leather and could not be polished. We were instructed how to drive military trucks. I easily passed the driver training course and was issued a military driver's license. Each of us was issued a footlocker placed at the end of our bunk.

After I had passed the driver's test, I took a shower but left my wallet with identification papers on top of my footlocker. When I returned the wallet was gone. I found it later with a few dollars, but without my papers. Because of that loss, I was not reissued a military driver's license, and for the rest of my Army duty never again drove a military vehicle.

All areas in the latrine were open – toilets, urinals, and showers. That loss of privacy was new for me. Latrine duty consisted of cleaning toilet bowls and urinals with a toothbrush. Lights were out at 9 p.m. sharp each night, with reveille (réveiller in French) at 5:30 each morning. A roll call was done each morning before breakfast. After eating, we tidied up our bunks and then fell in line to start the day's training at 7 a.m.

In mid-October, we had an overnight bivouac following a daylong march. We set up the 55-mm howitzers and fired them without using hearing protectors. Many of us had hearing loss by age 40 as a result of the very loud noise from these guns. We camped in pup tents that we carried, with a small tarp for the ground. We slept in our clothing and were issued only one wool blanket. It froze solid that night, dropping to 10 degrees F. It was a cold, uncomfortable experience, but nothing like what soldiers fighting in Europe had to endure, especially in the 1945 Battle of the Bulge in Belgium, during which a blizzard that lasted several days caused freezing toes and fingers. Many Germans fighting in the bitterly cold Russian winter of 1942–43 froze to death while trying to defecate in a snow bank with their pants pulled down.

We received $75 per month in pay, but we had little time for activities outside training. I did get involved in playing poker after the first and second paydays. Playing against card sharks, I had been dealt hands that often were second-high, and I lost two months in a row. I did little gambling after that despite opportunities to do so; even years afterward I never joined faculty colleagues on poker nights.

On trips to the PX (Post Exchange), I picked up needed supplies and occasionally beer. The language I learned in high school did not prepare me for the harsh language in the military. Most sentences in the Army

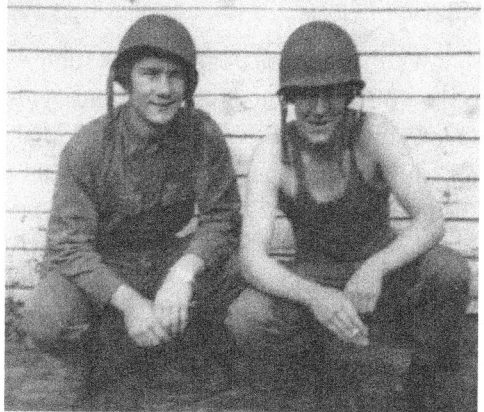

Private First Class Gordon Theilen, Fort Knox, Kentucky, October 1946.

included the f-word along with other swear words and slang. Scuttlebutt was present in everyday discussions that something or other was going to happen. It usually didn't, but most trainees learned to distrust the word of sergeants and officers, because most schedules were never followed.

Near the end of basic training, I was given an opportunity to investigate special forces training and assignment. Most of my high school friends at Fort Knox took assignments for overseas deployment. All went to Japan, including Ron Kamb, Rick Maisel, and Blair Smith. Dick McGranahan, Don Sagner, and I choose jump school at Fort Benning, Georgia. Dwayne McClendon was chosen to go OCS (Officer Candidate School), from which he graduated as a second lieutenant.

Paratrooper training, Fort Benning, Georgia

The Army Airborne Jump School consisted of 12 weeks of training to become disciplined paratroop soldiers. We marched double time, never walked. A fall safely from 12-foot platforms was the first step in learning to jump from a plane. In the next step, trainees were hoisted up 250-foot-high towers in open guided parachutes attached to cables, which enabled falling with a chute. Jumps out of a mock airplane with full parachute gear attached to a hookup cable provided training for real jumps. We were taught to exit the plane quickly so the entire group of jumpers would remain close together in order to easily assemble on the ground as a quick united fighting force.

We had a ride in an Army glider that was towed by a C-47 plane and released. These gliders were not efficient and mostly a disaster in combat, landing in rugged terrain, breaking apart and often killing most on board. We were given a choice of going into the glider unit or moving on to be jumpers. It was not a huge decision to decide against joining the 82nd Airborne Division glider unit, which was disbanded for obvious reasons in the late 1940s, before the Korean War began.

The night before my first jump, I went to a movie at the base theater. It was about spies and counterspies jumping out of a light bomber into enemy territory. The spy hookup cable was cut by the counterspy as he jumped, and the spy fell to his death. Wow, what a way to begin a career in the paratroopers service.

My first jump went well, but I had my eyes closed and did not open them until the chute opened. In 50 seconds I was on the ground. During the next four jumps, I had my eyes open and saw the tail of the C-46 as it went by and watched my chute open after a drop of 90 feet. Our jumps started at 1,200 feet and decreased in elevation until the last jump at 800 feet. We were required to complete five jumps to finish as qualified paratroopers and obtain jump wings, an emblem proudly worn on the left side of the chest.

We attached our rip cords to steel cables running the length of the interior of the plane. Troopers were taught to stand up all at the same time. The first sergeant would command, "Stand up, hook up, go!" and every trooper jumped out one after the other within just a few seconds, emptying the entire line of 16 men on each side of the plane (32 troopers in all).

As we jumped and the chute broke away from the ripcord, each of us yelled "Geronimo!" Each trooper wore an emergency chest chute. If properly used, the smaller emergency chute with a 24-foot canopy was hand fed out of the pack to insure opening without entangling with the failed streaming primary chute. There are many stories of jumpers becoming entangled with the failed chute. In certain combat jumps, such as during the retaking of Corregidor Island in the Philippines in 1945, jumpers in the 8th Airborne Division left the emergency chutes in the plane because the drop zone, surrounded by ocean, was so small, and the altitude of the plane was only 350 feet. Still, many jumpers drifted into the ocean and drowned.

During our training, landing within 45 to 50 seconds from a height of 800 to 1,200 feet meant the ground came up fast, with a few swings of the chute before hitting Earth like a 50-pound sack of potatoes and crumbling with the fall, as previously taught in jump school. The idea was that initial contact was to be made with the toes, followed by muscle masses touching ground. Knees, elbows, and the head were not to make contact.

Landing was never easy. On one occasion, my chute swung backward, making me hit the ground heels first. I fell backward on my buttocks and instantaneously hit the back of my head; I saw stars. It was daytime, not night. I had a sore head, neck, and buttocks for several days, but had to jump twice more in the next two days to obtain the paratrooper wings. I probably had a slight concussion, but medical evaluation was not even considered for such a hard landing impact.

On nice weather days, it was a beautiful sight to see all the chutes opening and falling to Earth. The ground and trees came closer and closer, almost like a blink of the eye. Our camouflaged green parachutes had canopies 28 feet in diameter with 36 cords (shrouds) on each side. Shrouds were made of 3/16-inch thick white braided nylon for added strength. Several thousand pounds of torque were required to break the shrouds, which were 12 feet long. The straps that went around each trooper's shoulders and waist were made of much thicker green nylon, about four inches wide and half an inch thick. The risers that held the 72 shroud cords above the shoulders extended a foot or so above my head and attached snugly to minimize discomfort during the sudden jolt when the chute opened. The planes traveled at 120 mph, and at that speed, a trooper fell 90 feet then suddenly stopped in the sky as the chute was free from the plane. If the harness rigging was not snug enough, the risers would snap the shoulders, resulting in "riser burns" with extreme bruising. Depending upon the severity, huge hematomas would develop.

On the day we completed jump school, a ceremony took place on the parade grounds, with troopers wearing well-pressed jump clothing and polished jump boots. Airborne troops were led to believe they were the best soldiers in the world and were told so every day of training. It was a form of brainwashing, and it worked. We were the best soldiers in the world.

Troopers were allowed to have their trouser pant legs tucked onto the top of their official-issue jump boots, the mark of an Airborne soldier. The tucked pant legs were held in place with rubber bands or condoms. The latter were freely issued to the troops to prevent them from contracting venereal diseases while on leave. Prostitutes were abundant near most army bases.

I spent my Christmas leave in Atlanta with George Taylor, a good friend from Downey in Southern California. We went to Christmas Eve services in a Lutheran church in Atlanta. I remember the minister greeting us, but no one else did. We would have welcomed an invitation to a home on Christmas Eve. The lack of hospitality never left my mind. Hundreds of times in the next several decades, I always attempted to greet strangers after church or in other places of community gathering. Reluctance to leave familiar territory to greet another person appears to be part of human nature. In animal behavior, it is referred to as territorial prerogative.

Racial discrimination

On a night leave, George and I attended a movie in Phenix City, Alabama, not far from Fort Benning. Phenix City was not subject to "Georgia blue laws" and we were able to buy alcoholic beverages and other goods that were not available in Georgia. When George and I got on the bus to come back to the base, an unforgettable incident occurred.

Racial segregation was still prevalent in the South in 1946, and seats in the back of the bus were designated for black people. On this particular evening, around 11:30 p.m., the black section on the last bus to leave town for the base was full, while the white section had several empty seats. A black sergeant and his wife got on and sat in the last row of the white section, next to the fully occupied black area, under the watchful gaze of the bus driver. The driver waited about 10 minutes for more passengers, but no one else boarded the bus. Finally, after a long delay and silence from everyone, the driver stood up and walked hurriedly toward the rear of the bus, stopped where the sergeant was sitting, and belligerently said in an extremely loud shout, "You black son-of-a-bitch, get back in the section where you belong."

The black couple were obviously from Detroit. The sergeant's wife told her husband, "Do not respond, this is not Detroit," and they went to the back of the bus and stood all the way back to the base. This was the epitome of following the letter of the law of that era rather than showing grace to a man serving his country in the Army. Such examples can explain the need for the civil rights movement that the Rev. Martin Luther King led. In all towns, public toilets were divided four ways: women, men, white, and black. The same applied for public drinking fountains, swimming pools, and other segregated facilities. It was also true in college and professional sports. Jackie Robinson was the first black athlete to play major league baseball, breaking the color barrier in baseball with the Brooklyn Dodgers after the team's manager, Branch Rickey, signed him. Robinson consequently went through trying times in his professional baseball career. I remembered the close friendship I had with my good friend, the Rev. LeRoy McGrew, and with other black high school classmates who did not regard skin color as a barrier to friendship. Bryan Brant, a black high-school classmate, became a minister and has traveled from New Jersey to attend several Richmond High School class of 1946 reunions.

After completing jump school training in February 1947, I was assigned to report at Camp Stoneman in Pittsburg, California, within two weeks for overseas shipment to the 8th Airborne in Japan. I hitched a ride home by flying from the air base at Fort Benning in a B-25 light bomber; I was the only passenger along with the pilot and co-pilot. We fueled somewhere in the Midwest, and while approaching the Rocky Mountains flew through an electrical storm that tossed the plane up and down several thousand feet at a time. The pilots took a rest and stopped overnight at an airbase near Phoenix. It was nice and warm in February in the Arizona desert. From here, we flew to Hamilton Air Force Base in Marin County. I hitchhiked to connect with a ferry crossing the San Francisco Bay from San Rafael to Richmond. It was good to be home after six months. The weather was spring-like and not wintry as it had been at Fort Benning. Most of my friends were gone except for my good girlfriend, Lorraine Johnson. We saw quite a bit of each other on my short visit, and I thought I had fallen back in love with her. I believe she felt the same way; however, it did not work out – a blessing in disguise.

82nd Airborne Division

Camp Stoneman was only 30 miles from Richmond. I arrived to find out that my orders had been changed from Hokkaido, Japan, with the 8th Airborne, to Fort Bragg, North Carolina, to join the famous 82nd Airborne Division. I took a passenger train to Fort Bragg, where I arrived several days later.

I was assigned to Special Regiment Company, and for the next year I packed and repaired parachutes daily. The 82nd Airborne Division was spit and polish and double-time on movement. The first sergeant would yell, "Double-time soldiers!" We were extremely fit and ready for combat at a minute's notice.

For each parachute that I packed, I made an entry in a ledger book with the date and my name as packer. All chutes had to be repacked within 60 days of the previous packing. The packing shed was a long structure that accommodated a dozen or so packing tables. A chute was placed on a table and attached at the round open portion of the canopy, a foot in diameter. This allowed air to go through the chute to prevent it from collapsing during a jump. If the shroud lines were tangled or knotted, we untangled them. We had to maintain tension on the shrouds while packing. I would grip the lines between my fingers, fold the chute neatly, and then stack it from the front of the canopy to fit snugly into the pack. We were expected to finish packing a chute within three to four minutes.

I was required to serve guard duty frequently, at times assigned to guard the base prison. Guard duty required carrying a loaded rifle and walking back and forth around the prison woven wired fence topped with concertina wire. Soldiers within had been sentenced to terms ranging from a month to as much as a year, usually for minor offenses. A soldier who was convicted of a major crime served a minimum sentence of one year of hard labor at a maximum-security military prison, such as the one at Fort Leavenworth, Kansas. Many were sentenced to five years and longer, depending upon the crime.

Cleveland Indians and Philadelphia Athletics

I was awarded a three-day pass for being the best-groomed solider and maintaining the best-kept barracks cot. I hitched by plane from Fort Bragg to southern Illinois, then by car and train to Cleveland to visit uncle Ray Schaller, his wife Alice, and their baby boy, Dale. Ray took me to see the Cleveland Indians play the Philadelphia Athletics. Connie Mack, famous owner of the Athletics, actively managed the team in advanced old age. Dressed in a suit and tie, he directed fielders by waving his arms one way or another to move a player's position when a certain Indians batter would come to the plate. I saw famous Indians pitcher Bob Feller pitch a winning game. It was a real thrill. I equate seeing that game with inheriting the same algebra book Lefty Gomez had years before me in high school.

I followed the San Francisco Giants even before they came to San Francisco in 1956 and remember when Bobby Thompson's walk-off home run snatched the National League Championship for the Giants as they beat the Dodgers. Announcer Russ Hodges' call of that home run was repeated over and over: "The Giants win the pennant! The Giants win the pennant! The Giants win the pennant, and they're going crazy!" The dramatic game-winning three-run homer off of Thompson's bat that October day in 1951 came to be known as "the shot heard 'round the world." I listened to that call live on my car radio in the parking lot of the UC Davis Chemistry Building. It was an unforgettably memorable moment in my 75 years as a Giants fan.

I returned to Washington, D.C., by train and from there hitchhiked by plane to Fort Bragg. Upon my return, I was assigned to a special Airborne demonstration group assigned to visit various Army posts to discuss what the Airborne does. I presented demonstrations at Fort Leavenworth near Manhattan, Kansas, and Fort Sill, Oklahoma. I received a personal letter signed by the

HEADQUARTERS 82ND AIRBORNE DIVISION
OFFICE OF THE DIVISION COMMANDER

AADCG 201.22

Fort Bragg, N.C.
30 January 1948

SUBJECT: Letter of Appreciation

THRU: Commanding Officer, 82d Airborne Parachute Maintenance Company, 82d Airborne Division, Fort Bragg, N. C.

TO: Technician Fourth Grade Gordon H. Theilen, 82d Airborne Parachute Maintenance Company, 82d Airborne Division, Fort Bragg, North Carolina

1. I have received personal letters from Major General White, Commandant at the Ground General School, Fort Riley, Kansas and Colonel Sears, Assistant Commandant of the Armored School, Fort Knox, Kentucky, expressing appreciation for and commending very highly the conduct, presentation of the display, attitude, military appearance and knowledge of subjects shown by the Airborne Demonstration Team which visited those stations on the 9th and 12th of January 1948. I have learned too, that the team made a very fine impression while at Fort Leavenworth.

2. As a member of this team, your performance reflects credit upon you and the 82d Airborne Division. I am pleased to add my appreciation for your personal contribution to the over-all showing of the team and thank you for a job well done.

JAMES M. GAVIN
Major General, USA
Commanding

Letter from General Jumpin' Jim Gavin.

Division two-star General, "Jumpin' Jim" Gavin, who complimented me on my participation and on comments that accompanying officers had made about me. I was a staff sergeant grade three and pleased to be recognized for doing an outstanding job. Those talks I gave on the benefits and advantages of being in the Airborne marked the beginning of my teaching career.

Back at the base, Gen. Gavin came to the jump field from his office every week and jumped with enlisted soldiers. He introduced himself on one of those occasions, giving me the opportunity to meet a leading World War II hero. In order to maintain jump status, troopers had to jump every three months. I was often at the jump field during these practice jumps, making sure all was in order with jumpers' parachutes.

Gen. Gavin began his army career as a private and went to Officer Candidate School to become an officer. In the 82nd Airborne Division campaign that took place in 1944 in Sicily, our Navy mistakenly shot down several of the 82nd Airborne Division planes carrying combat soldiers. Bird Colonel (top-ranking colonel) Gavin was promoted to one-star brigadier general in Sicily, becoming the youngest major general in the U.S. Army. He had a meritorious career and was a soldier's general. He was always out front with his division, a rarity among military leaders regardless of time in history. There have been a few others, such as Stonewall Jackson, general in the confederate army; Gen. George Patton; and on the enemy side in World War II, Field Marshal Erwin Rommel.

Jumping Jim was the only one who I personally knew. The closest I came to Stonewall Jackson and Rommel was their graves. Rommel was buried in his home village, Herrlingen near Ulm, Germany. I was with Dr. Otto Straub, a veterinary friend, in 1962 traveling to the World Veterinary Conference in Hanover. Along the way we went by Herrlingen, where Rommel was buried, and we went to see the grave. Years later on a few occasions I stopped with others who wished to see Rommel's grave.

I made the best of military life and had good experiences to remember, but military life has few freedoms in comparison with those of civilians. My 18 months of service constituted valuable experience with authoritative demands.

Discharge and return to Richmond

Following my discharge on February 16, 1948, I traveled to Minnesota and visited with my Schaller grandparents and relatives in the Maynard area, and with Theilen grandparents in the Le Mars area. George Taylor, a friend of mine from the 82nd Airborne, was discharged a bit later. George had purchased a used 1940 Ford two-door passenger sedan in Baltimore and drove from there to Iowa to meet me. We visited with some of his relatives near Dallas, Texas, and then followed U.S. 66 through Amarillo, Tucumcari, Albuquerque, Kingman, Barstow, San Bernardino to its end near Los Angeles. I have often relived this trip by listening to the classic Bobby Troup song "(Get Your Kicks On) Route 66."

Commencing in 1993 and several times thereafter, I traveled the new Interstate 40, crossing many of the same places in a Ford three-quarter-ton pickup truck with a gooseneck hitch towing a converted stock trailer filled

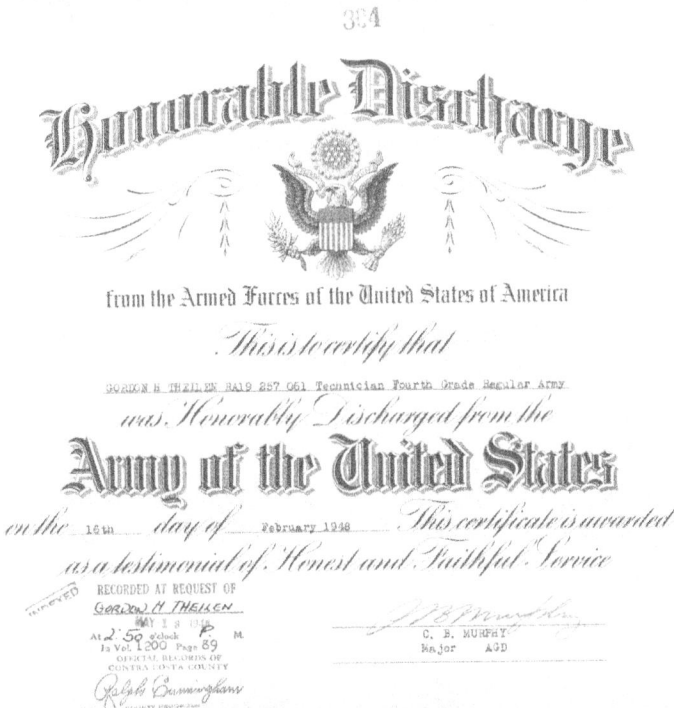

A valued document – Honorable Discharge certificate, February 16, 1948.

111

with dogs and horses. These trips were to attend field trials in the Midwest and the American Brittany Club's national competitions in Booneville, Arkansas. The Boy With the Wounded Thumb participated in field-trialing Brittany dogs off horseback from 1987 unto 2010. The goal in these activities was always to go to the extreme limit of testing my ability to achieve with a field placement for one of my dogs, even if the field endeavor seemed at the beginning nearly impossible to achieve a placement. My life was filled with curiosity and wonder about what was possible.

On my return to Richmond following my discharge from military service, I resumed work at the Standard Oil Refinery, from March until the start of summer session at the University of California, Berkeley, in June 1948. It was good to be home and see former high school friends, both male and female. But changes were occurring. Although the Standard Oil refinery still produced familiar odors, three shipyards were closing down. No longer did we hear the sound of "Rosie the Riveter" working away within hearing range of our home. The moist evening air used to enhance the noise and carry sound in a way that made us feel like being at the shipyard itself, even though it was two and a half miles away.

I also landed a job with a body and fender shop on San Pablo Avenue just before the El Cerrito city limits. I removed damaged fenders and other damaged parts, and repaired or replaced fenders and hoods. I sanded rusted metal, readying it for priming and final painting in the paint room. I was fortunate to get the job, which became part-time after I started classes at the UC Berkeley. The owner was a native of Minnesota, from a town not far from where I used to live, and he knew relatives of mine in the Maynard, Clara City and Montevideo regions.

Richmond had been semirural when we first moved there, but that changed rapidly when the population exploded during World War II and the environment changed to one that no longer embraced societal civility. The apartment buildings constructed in south Richmond during the war years were rapidly becoming rundown, as the money made available to build and maintain them during wartime no longer was available. The community that inhabited them during the postwar era was relatively lawless, with a huge increase in crime. Richmond no longer was the typical middle-class city it had once been, and it never recovered from the rapid growth and emerging ethnic change that occurred during the war years. Many moved from Richmond and relocated in communities east of San Pablo Avenue, the dividing line between gradual and eventually huge societal changes.

Richmond further deteriorated in the last three decades of the 20th century. The high school became a building with barred windows, with a surrounding cyclone fence, in a community with little respect for education, law, and order. Similar change came to cities all around the Bay Area, from Vallejo to Pinole, Albany, Berkeley, Oakland, Alameda, San Jose, and San Francisco. Socioeconomic change occurred despite President Roosevelt's New Deal and President Johnson's Great Society. It impacted most of my high-school friends, and few remained in the changed city after graduation. Re-establishing the family unit and taking seriously the Ten Commandments and commitment to honor God are formulas for improved social exchange.

CHAPTER 14

University Education at UC Berkeley

"A light from the shadows shall spring."
– John Ronald Reuel Tolkien

Freshman

Upon my return to civilian life in March 1948, my goal was to begin a college education in preparation for a degree in veterinary medicine. I enrolled in my first college classes in the summer session at the University of California, Berkeley. I was on probation as a full-time student until I completed Subject A, "Bonehead English," which I did not pass in high school. At UC Berkeley, I achieved a passing grade and became a fully qualified student. Ms. Byrnes, my high school English Subject A teacher, would have been amazed, as she advised me against trying to attend the University of California because my verbal and writing skills were insufficient. She did not have a clue that since the age of 5, I was determined to be a university-educated veterinarian.

Attending summer-session classes helped me make the transition from high school to college quizzes and exams. The individualized help that high-school teachers had given me no longer was available. Attending Chemistry IA, IB and other classes with a class size of a thousand was at first overwhelming. However, labs were smaller, and lab assistants helped students individually.

I had little opportunity to develop friendships in the large classroom settings, but I did make friends at the Sigma Chi fraternity. I commuted from my parents' home in Richmond, and most of my close friends were former high-school acquaintances who had become members of Sigma Chi. They included Dick Macfie, Dwayne McClendon, and Dick McGranahan. I developed other good fraternity friends, including Bo Phillips and Paul Jacobs from Dixon. Dick McGranahan left school due to alcoholism, which led eventually to a failed life and early death from substance abuse. The other Jolly Boys from high school remained alive well into their 80s. The next to die was Ernie Liebhardt in 2014, followed by Dwayne in 2015, and Dick Macfie in 2016.

I was best man at Dick Macfie and Lil Sernack's wedding, and they have remained our very dear friends. Hands down, my best friend was Dick Macfie. I was in the wedding party for Dwayne and Trudy McClendon. Trudy died in her late 40s from cancer. Dwayne remarried, and remained a good friend of mine for decades.

I drove back and forth from Richmond to UC Berkeley in a 1940 two-door Ford sedan. Parking areas on the north side of campus were closer to classes than parking at the fraternity house on the south side, a mile away. My arrangement to live at home helped save enough money for my eventual transfer to UC Davis and its veterinary school.

In autumn 1948 and 1949, I attended exciting football games. Cal had teams coached by Pappy Waldorf, and he coached the Golden Bears to the Rose Bowl on New Year's Day 1949 (playing against opponent Northwestern), 1950 (against Ohio State), and 1951 (Michigan). Attending that game against Big 10 Northwestern was a real thrill, even though Cal lost that day. In 1949 I began dating Ruth Ann Fox, a relationship that continued until I transferred to UC Davis. She attended the University of the Pacific and became involved in campus activities, which led to her meeting and marrying a classmate. Before Ruth Ann, I had dated Lucille Mallan quite seriously. Lucille and I were extremely good friends, but going out with Ruth Ann brought dates with Lucille to an end. Lucille and I have remained good friends for decades.

During my first one and half years at UC Berkeley as a pre-veterinary major, I did well academically, attaining an overall B average. Admittance to veterinary school depended on high scholastic achievement, animal experience, and a strong desire to become a veterinarian. In addition to my background as a farm boy until the age of 11, I had worked for Dr. Seymour Roberts in high school and Dr. Robert Walker, primarily a farm-animal practitioner, while in college.

Learning to 'read' animals

The Boy With the Wounded Thumb was determined not just to qualify for admission to vet school, but to make a mark in the field. "Gordon, when you become a veterinarian, be sure to do something that no other has done," Dr. Seymour Roberts said while I was working for him. He was a remarkable man, and working with him I learned special aspects of veterinary medicine with desire to initiate something professionally special.

To initiate new concepts, a person needs vision and curiosity with no fear of failure. Men and women well known in various walks of life are those who have stuck with visions and curiosities. Such recognized persons in cancer medicine included Vilhelm Ellermann and Oluf Bang, who discovered the cause of chicken leukemia in 1902; Peyton Rous, who discovered chicken sarcoma in 1910; Katsusaburo Yamagiwa and Koichi Ichikawa, who discovered the first chemical cause of cancer in 1915; and Ludwig Gross, discovered first mouse leukemia virus in 1955.

In the summer of 1949, after my first year at the university, I began working as an unpaid volunteer for Dr. Bob Walker, who had a mixed large- and small-animal veterinary practice in Pleasanton. His emphasis was on farm animals, whereas Dr. Roberts had been primarily a veterinarian for pet animals. Dr. Walker was scholastically the top of his graduating class at Washington State Veterinary School, where he finished in 1945 as a Phi Beta Kappa. He was a very bright and learned veterinarian, and working with him taught me new aspects of veterinary medicine and ways to "read" large animals. However, I also learned by observing him that a person under pressure should not lose his temper or fail to keep a level mind. It became obvious that inability to keep a level head while working under pressure would result in a dysfunctional veterinary career.

Pressures of veterinary practice

Dr. Walker was a workaholic who often skipped breakfast and, for lunch, would rush into the house, pour a glass of red wine, crack two eggs into it, and drink it down within a minute. He maintained a very busy pace from early in the morning to late at night. After the quick, unusual lunchtime nourishment, he would be on his way again to take farm calls. I often went with him on afternoon calls and would help bring drugs and equipment from the car to the animal that needed examination and treatment. I spent mornings cleaning kennels and taking phone calls from ranchers and farmers who needed a veterinarian. In the afternoon, Mrs. Walker would take the calls. Her husband would call his office from the ranch where he was treating an animal, and she would tell him where to go next.

One day on a dairy farm, we attended to a cow that had given birth a few days before and had a retained placenta. I had brought the water and detergent needed for cleanliness to remove the placenta, as Dr. Walker did something else and continued talking with the farmer. As I waited for him, he said, "Gordon aren't you going to pick up the tail so I can wash the cow's vulva and bring out the hanging placenta?" I answered, "I was waiting for you," and he replied, "you are to anticipate my every move."

That made me realize that Dr. Walker was short on patience. I was a volunteer working for experience, not pay. I slept on a cot in a horse stable with a dirt floor and no screens. Every morning, I could hardly open my eyes due to mosquito or spider bites. Often in evenings, after a dinner I ate with the family, I would babysit the two young children, about 2 and 4 years old, so the Walkers could go out for some relaxation. When Bob and his wife were away, I answered the phone and took messages about clients needing veterinary service. I was determined to gain the experience needed for admission into veterinary school despite the living conditions and expectations. Dr. Walker's personality troubled me, as I did not see him taking enjoyment in what he was doing. His life was rushed and seemingly without joy or faith. He needed to find some balance.

The balanced triad: An axiom on professional life

I received word in 1954 that Dr. Walker, a veterinarian with many attributes, had committed suicide. Years later, while preparing a lecture for an oncology class, I had a flashback to Dr. Walker and what might have been if only he had led a balanced professional life. I wanted to illustrate that life consists of more than just veterinary medicine, and I devised a diagram that was subtly based on Christian faith. I titled it "A Balanced Triad." I made up one slide to project during the last lecture in the quarter. I labeled the tip of the triangle "Family and Friends," the right corner "Hobbies and Extracurricular" and the left corner "Professional Activities." In the center I wrote "Faith," and captioned the diagram "An axiom on a successful professional life."

I told students they should try to carry out life's commitments with balancing main facets. I became known as the "Triad Professor." Some students said they had time only to study and not for much else. Dr. Walker had little time for anything other than his practice. His suicide left a big impression on me, and ever since I have tried to guide persons into a balanced, productive, and enjoyable life by leaning on God for guidance. He gave His only begotten son that we would be saved if by faith we accepted Christ's death on the cross and resurrection as our propitiation for Salvation and everlasting life.

Figure 1: Balanced Triad

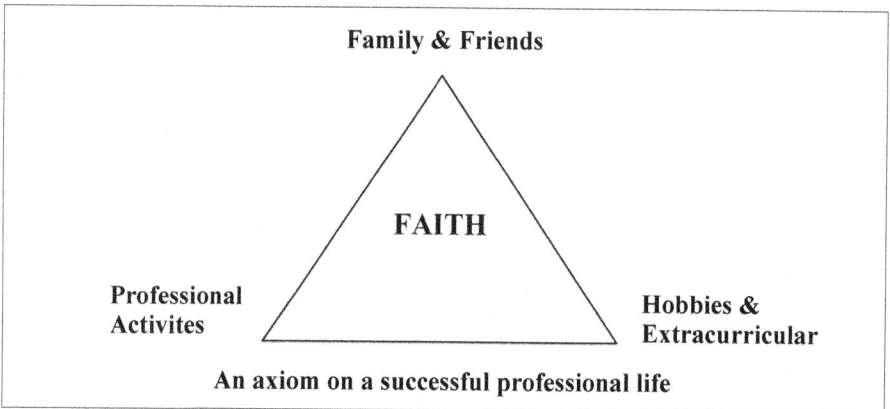

Family & Friends

FAITH

Professional
Activites

Hobbies &
Extracurricular

An axiom on a successful professional life

The curse of suicide

Several colleagues and friends of mine have committed suicide. Of three that occurred in Davis, the most tragic was that of Larry McFarland, a 41-year-old veterinary school professor who attended a committee meeting on a Friday afternoon with me in April 1972. When we parted, I said, "Larry, have a good weekend." He seemed fine, but he had recently separated from his wife and was residing alone in an apartment. Around 11 p.m. that evening, he went to the house where his wife and three teenage children lived. The children were out for Friday night festivities. When they came home, he murdered them and his wife, set the house on fire, and killed himself – because his wife had left him for another man. He was distraught over the separation and was unwilling to live separately from them.

Sometime later, a neighbor teenage boy, Howard Kasamatis, was home from college for Christmas vacation. I saw him in front of his home as I was returning from a Friday evening bike ride in a dense December fog. His parents and the family were good friends and fellow members of Davis Lutheran Church. I wished Howard a good Christmas holiday and we parted. That evening, he hung himself in a backyard tree. Kas, his father, found him the next morning dangling from a tree limb on a side of the house rarely used in the winter months.

On another Friday afternoon in October 1980, veterinary Professor John Kendrick met me in a UC Davis hallway as both of us were going home for the evening. He asked me if I would meet with one of his graduate students who was studying a virus in the area of my expertise. I said surely. That evening, John took an overdose of barbiturates in the bathtub. He was living in a second-floor apartment, and water from the overflowing tub in which he drowned dripped through the ceiling to the apartment below. He, too, had just separated from his wife and a family of several children, some of college age. John was only 56 years old when he died. Years later, one of his sons also committed suicide.

Alice Rodgers lived on the east side of Pitt School Road, just north of Dixon and across the road from Jim Fulmore's dairy farm, on which Ray and Doreen Simon, my future in-laws, lived. The Simons were good friends with Alice, who had been separated from her physically abusive husband, Nate. Jim Rodgers, Alice and Nate's oldest son, committed a murder-suicide just as Larry McFarland had. Jim shot his wife, their three young children and then himself; the motive likewise was that his wife had left him and taken the children.

These suicides and the difficulties encountered by other students, friends, and colleagues who had drug and alcohol problems led to development of the balanced triad concept, which I related to students for the last 10 years of my teaching career. I do not know how much of a difference my lectures had. My goal was to impress upon my students that professional life must be balanced in order to avoid real personal problems.

UC Davis

In the summer of 1949, I visited the University of California, Davis. A college fraternity friend, Paul Jacobs, told me I should visit his Dixon High School classmate, Carolyn Simon, who worked in the soda fountain at the Queensbury Pharmacy on First Street, just south of A Street in Dixon. I stopped by, Carolyn and I had a pleasant visit, and I ordered a chocolate-malt milkshake that was the best I ever tasted. I again saw Carolyn when I transferred to UC Davis in January of 1950. She worked part-time in the co-op serving coffee and sandwiches as a freshman at UC Davis. We saw each other occasionally, but there was no overt action on my part to ask her for a date because I was seriously connected at the time with Ruth Ann Fox.

I had difficulty at first cutting my strings to UC Berkeley because of strong friendships in the Sigma Chi fraternity and special friends, including Dick Macfie, Dwayne McClendon and Bo Phillips, as well as friends in Richmond and church membership at Trinity Lutheran on Barrett and 19th streets. I also missed the Bay Area climate, the cool ocean breezes, and even the fog, particularly in summer months. Davis, in the Sacramento Valley, has a hot summer climate.

West Hall

Adaptation to new surroundings and friends often occurs slowly, but after a few months at UC Davis, my life became as memorable as my high school days, and much more memorable than attending UC Berkeley. I lived on the third floor of West Hall, a wooden dormitory that had been built in 1914. I had terrific roommates, Clayton Finch and Ed Nevin, and I became exceptionally good friends with them and with others in West Hall and elsewhere on campus. Dorm life did not have the rituals of a fraternity, but solid, lifelong friendships developed. As warm spring weather came along, many water fights took place, and the hallways often were running with water. On weekends there were beer parties at Putah Creek, from which students would come back inebriated.

On one occasion, I had gone to the library to study away from the hubbub of students having all sorts of fun. When I went back my room, Clayton was there as Ed returned from a beer party feeling no pain. Just before he entered the room, a multitude of firecrackers went off very nearby – some of them just outside our door. Then a knock came at the door and Ed yelled, "Who in the hell is it?"

"Campus police."

Ed went to the door and the officer said, "Have you been letting off firecrackers or know who has?" Ed, slurring his words, said "Firerrr crackerrrs? I haven't heard any go off."

The officer was standing almost ankle deep in spent firecracker paper. The situation ended with warnings rather than bookings. Ed was not an alcoholic, and became a successful Southern California practicing veterinarian. Clayton became a well-known grain broker. Most of my fellow students achieved leadership roles in their areas of endeavor. The enjoyment of living as students was part and parcel of becoming a complete human being and responsible citizen who would contribute meaningfully to communities all over the United States and many places elsewhere in the world.

We were fed a lot of beans in the cafeteria, and, needless to say, fellow students did a lot of farting. Ed Nevin, Bill Priester, Clayton Finch, Stan Feidel, and others would sit on their cots, light a match, hold it near their butts, and let loose. Flames would spew out like a miniature standpipe burning off gas at the Standard Oil Refinery, where I had worked not too long before. No one was ever burned, but it looked quite likely at times. This activity went beyond the saying you are a "swell, fart-smelling person."

Everyone was perpetually on the lookout for a prank waiting to happen. The dorms had no air-conditioning, and in warm weather windows were always open. Toilets and showers for each floor accommodated about 40 students each.

The campus was small, and most academic buildings faced the block-square "quad." The lawn was a bit sunken to enable irrigation flooding of the grass in the summer; the entire quad was lined with cork oak trees that had significance for me. UC Davis was strictly an agricultural campus in the early 1950s, and hundreds of acres of cropland surrounded the campus.

Campus facilities included animal husbandry barns and pastures for dairy cattle, sheep, hogs, horses, poultry, and bee keeping. It was like living on a huge farm, and made the Boy With the Wounded Thumb feel that he was revisiting the Minnesota farms of his childhood. The atmosphere was so much more endearing than that at UC Berkeley, which had seemed huge and impersonal.

Class sizes at UC Davis were smaller than at UC Berkeley, and friendships developed easily. In 1950, the Davis campus had only 1,500 students, 150 of them women. For reasons I do not recall, I began to become interested in Carolyn. The main reason, I suspect, was the breakup and severing ties with Ruth Ann. It was difficult at first to get a date with Carolyn because she had dates lined up weeks ahead of time.

In the summer of 1950, Carolyn had gone with her family to visit relatives on the island of Jersey in the Channel Islands off the coast of France. That summer, I worked for Sacramento Hereford Ranch in West Sacramento owned by the Richard family. The cattle were raised specially for show competition at county and state fairs. I did not obtain the type of animal experience I felt I needed, quit the job and was hired by the manager of the Heather Farm, a Thoroughbred racehorse farm near Walnut Creek. I learned a tremendous amount about horse husbandry, and the manager, an expert in horse dentistry, taught me skills I utilized throughout a good part of my veterinary career. While working there, I became acquainted with a fine, dark bay-colored Thoroughbred stud horse, Soleil De Midi. It was a pleasant job that served me well for years to come.

When Carolyn returned, she continued her classes at UC Davis, intending to transfer to UC Berkeley in the spring semester of 1951. However, she developed pneumonia and was hospitalized in the UC Davis student health care center for several days. I visited with her frequently, and when she was released, our dating began on a causal basis. It became serious enough that she decided to complete her degree in Home Economics at UC Davis. Once the love bug hit, we got together every weekend. This close relationship expanded when she invited me to a Sadie Hawkins dance on February 29, 1952 at the old Recreation Hall located where the Freeborn Hall auditorium now stands. (Sadie Hawkins Day was a pseudo-holiday that originated in Al Capp's classic hillbilly comic strip "Li'l Abner." This inspired Sadie Hawkins dances, to which girls asked boys out.) I took Carolyn home for the weekend at her parents' home off Pitt School Road, about two miles north of Dixon. In gentlemanly fashion, I took her to the door, where, for the first time, we had a goodnight kiss. This started a real spark – similar, I suspect, to the sparks created by the fireflies I first observed in 1942 at Detroit Lakes, Minnesota.

By the summer of 1952 we were dating seriously. I occasionally had seen her in 1951 while working at Harvey McDougal Cattle Feedlot at Collinsville, about 30 miles south of Dixon.

McDougal Feedlot

The McDougal Feedlot was a facility that fed several thousand cattle at one time. Yearling cattle coming off the range would be placed in a pen accommodating several hundred head. They would be fed a mixture of concentrate to induce a weight gain of four pounds per day. The starting weight would be 700 pounds, and market weight would range from 1,100 to 1,300 pounds. Thus, at a four pounds weight gain per day, the yearling cattle would be in the field lot four to five months.

Occasionally, a heifer coming off the range would be with calf and give birth. The calf would be killed. On two occasions, a calf was given to me and one was raised by Col. Lyman Phillips, the father of Bo Phillips, a Sigma Chi fraternity brother from Cal. The Phillips ranch was located near Dixon. The other calf was raised by Carolyn's father, on his dairy farm north of Dixon. When raised, these beef cattle provided a good quantity of meat for poor students like ourselves.

Work at the McDougal Feedlot started at 5:30 a.m. after getting up at 4:30 a.m. to eat breakfast in the employee mess hall. About 25 of us lived at the facility, ate in the mess and slept in the bunkhouse. I performed many tasks, starting with the weekly cleaning of water tanks. This entailed draining the concrete basins, scrubbing them out with a brush on a handle, and refilling them with water. As I entered each pen of about an acre in size, 250 head of cattle would run toward me and investigate me as an intruder in their territory. They never were hostile unless a young heifer had been bred at an early age and given birth to a calf. Cows after giving birth are extremely protective of their newborn.

Feedlot odor is different from all other animal odors. It is a mixture of cattle manure, dust (or mud in winter), and concentrated feed (which at this lot contained beet pulp with an extremely potent odor all its own), intermixed with freshly ground hay and grains of various types. Such feed odors mixed with the aromas of manure and dust leaves sensory memories not forgotten. I recall these odors every time I drive south through California on Interstate 5 and pass the Harris Ranch feedlot near Coalinga.

Dick McDougal and I bucked hay during the annual harvest. These were five-wire bales weighing 225 pounds each. After an eight-hour day of stacking bales ("bucking hay") several levels high on a hay truck, fellow workers and I were ready to hit the sack right after dinner, only to arise at 4:30 a.m. and go again until several thousand acres of hay had been hauled to the hay barn.

I also drove a feed truck that mixed and hauled feed consisting of hay, beet pulp and many varieties of grains. The beet pulp added nutrients as well as moisture and succulence to the feed. The feed mix was extremely high in protein, fat and TDN (total digestible nutrients). The truck had a spout extending from the feed tank. A worker called a "feeder" stood on a platform next to the feed tank and controlled the amount of feed needed for each pen. This was a science, and the cattle in each pen received an amount of feed calculated to maintain a daily weight gain of four pounds. Today, feeding cattle is calculated by computer and the amount is automatically delivered.

Feedlot science is an aspect of veterinary medicine in which cattle are treated as a herd, not as individuals. The animals were processed through cattle chutes to squeeze chutes for vaccinations, and when ready for market were pushed through other chutes to be loaded onto cattle trucks to go to slaughter. Electric prods were used to keep resistant animals moving along through the chutes. There was no feeling of compassion for the individual animal, only daily feeding and water to maintain a needed weight gain. There was a feeling that cattle were imprisoned. Cattle had no protection from the hot sun or from the evening Sacramento River Delta winds. Daily temperatures in summer fluctuated from the low 60s at night to the high 90s in the day. In winter, the lots were extremely muddy, and cattle stayed on mounds of dirt mixed with manure to stay warm.

CHAPTER 15

Proposal and Marriage

"Alone we can do so little, together we can do much."
– Helen Keller

Carolyn and I had fallen in love when she invited me to the Sadie Hawkins Dance. After that, we never again showed affection for another person to date or love. I proposed to her following a period of anticipation with an extra-special event in mind. I had an inner good feeling about eating a meal in the City by the Bay. San Francisco had been a nostalgic location since my first visit in 1939, when attending the Golden Gate International Exposition on Treasure Island shortly after leaving the Midwest. October was the month that best fit proposal plans with good weather and no rain or fog. The anticipated site was Bay overlook at Coit Tower, the slender white column structure rising from Telegraph Hill with a spectacular view of glistening San Francisco Bay on a night lit by a harvest full moon.

San Francisco always has been known for wonderful restaurants and ethnic cuisines, notably in a neighborhood known around the world as Chinatown. As a high-school student, Chinese food on Friday nights with six classmates, the Jolly Boys, was special when we ate in Chinatown. But for this special proposal evening in 1952, I favored German food. I had been partial to German food, which is what my grandparents mostly ate, since my boyhood in Minnesota,

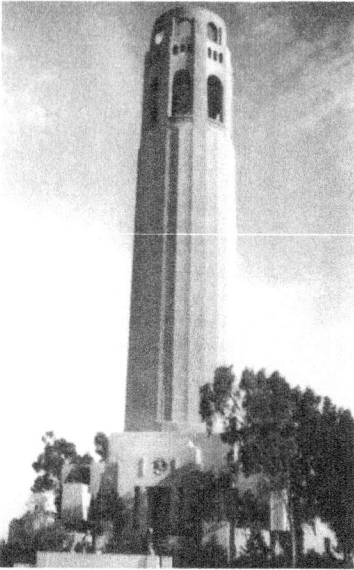

Coit Tower in San Francisco.

but Carolyn was unfamiliar with German cuisine.

We had dinner at The Shadows, a well-known German restaurant on Montgomery Street. Pickled pigs feet was an appetizer, followed by a main course of beef with traditional gravy, sauerkraut, and vegetables on the side. Soft cookies served with ice cream and apple strudel satisfied the palate.

Afterward, my sweetheart and I went to Coit Tower in North Beach. We walked up Telegraph Hill from Filbert Street, on steps lined by beautiful flowers, to the terraces of Pioneer Park at the base of the tower. At this location, 275 feet above sea level, a windmill-like structure known as a semaphore had been erected in 1850 to "telegraph" the rest of the city, by means of adjustable arms on a pole, what kind of ships and cargo were headed into port. The system was dismantled in 1852 with the arrival of the electric telegraph, but the name Telegraph Hill remained. Coit Tower wasn't completed until 1933, but Pioneer Park, established atop the hill in 1879 to celebrate the nation's centennial, had immediately become one of the city's most celebrated vista points.

From the park terrace high above the city, we could see the gorgeous full moon with its craters and reflecting light on the bay, the graceful swoops of the Golden Gate and Bay bridges, and a sea of lights twinkling all around us. It was the perfect environment for marriage proposal.

The Boy With the Wounded Thumb asked Carolyn to marry him, and she replied "yes." There was a warm embrace and kiss, and then I gave her my Sigma Chi fraternity pin as an engagement symbol in place of the traditional ring, for which I had little money to purchase.

A warm courtship followed, during which time we came to know each other's likes and dislikes. Carolyn, being a dairyman's daughter, and I, originally a farm boy, obviously liked country living and the out-of-doors.

During our courtship before proposal, Carolyn had lived on the third floor of South Hall at UC Davis and I on the third floor of West Hall. Both were on the quad at the center of campus. We would see each other nightly after the campus library closed at 11 p.m. Carolyn had a part-time job at the delicatessen in Rec Hall, which closed a half-hour later. We would have a cup of coffee and say good night until the next night. On our way back to the dorms, we often climbed the cork-oak trees that lined the quad.

We were married March 6, 1953, at All Saints Episcopal Church in Carmel-by-the-Sea on the coast. Two weeks earlier, when we were on our way to make arrangements before the wedding, a law enforcement officer pulled me over in Morgan Hill for going 45 miles per hour in a 30-mile zone. On our way to Carmel for our wedding on March 6, I stopped by City Hall and was able to speak with the traffic judge. I asked him to dismiss my fine as a wedding present, and the genie of good fortune was present. The case was dismissed. It was good fortune indeed, because we were in need of every penny we could muster to provide for food and shelter.

Those in attendance at the wedding were Carolyn's parents, Ray and Doreen Simon; her older brother, Mike Simon; his wife Mary; my parents, Lou and Ema Theilen; and my sister, Blythe, was maid of honor, and Carolyn's younger brother, Phil, was best man. Blythe played the Lord's Prayer on her violin. At our 62nd wedding anniversary at Trinity Free Lutheran in Dixon she again played the Lord's Prayer, a wonderful reminder of our wedding day.

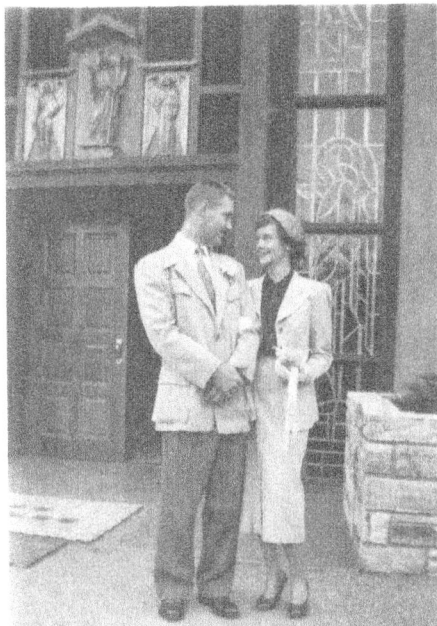

Carolyn and me after our wedding on March 6, 1953.

Ray hosted a memorable reception at the Highlands Inn with a wonderful meal. Carolyn and I spent our short honeymoon in Carmel and the Big Sur coastal area, where we stayed in a cabin secluded in the wonderful redwood forest. We had a small platter turnstile record player, and listened to six platters over and over. They included Puccini's *Madame Butterfly* with the opera star singing *La Bohème* as part of the repertoire.

Phil loaned us his new 1951 yellow Ford convertible. We certainly enjoyed driving California Highway 1 along the coast with the top down. The weather was especially gorgeous for early March. Upon our return to Davis, we stayed a few days with Ray and Doreen before moving in for a few months with a UC Davis professor who lived in the Willowbank neighborhood of Davis.

The first life-changing event upon return from our honeymoon was giving our cigarettes away. On March 9, 1953, both of us quit smoking, never again to use tobacco products in our 63 years and counting of married life. Besides saving us from a host of medical problems later in life, the money saved from buying cigarettes helped keep us in food and purchase gas for our car, a 1939 two-door Plymouth sedan that was a gift from my parents, who had purchased it in 1942.

At the time we were married, I was a junior in veterinary school. My grades were average up to the time of marriage, but after that they improved. In my fourth-year assessment, I ranked among the top in clinical medicine. After graduation, I began a short career in private practice in Tillamook, Oregon.

Carolyn and I became an adaptable couple, never regretting God's gift of a loving and sharing marriage and joining each other as "one flesh" – Matthew 19:6. In our advanced age, many have asked about our secret to a successful life together. My instant reply: "God sent an angel to Earth on June 21, 1931, and she became my bride." Carolyn always has been there for me, and has been an extraordinary helpmate. We have equally and openly discussed our needs and desires and found solutions together. We agreed to abide by each other in directing and raising our three children. We had no favorites and tried to have the children equally receive gifts and favors.

We enjoyed family vacations, educational growth, and discussing politics and Christian faith together. We never had a major misunderstanding, and over six decades of our marriage, Carolyn never complained about what I was doing wrong or that she was being singled out for suffering multiple sclerosis for 40 years. I can unequivocally say that she was largely responsible for professional successes. She has been a joy to share life, leaving no desire to have another sexual relationship or an intimate female friendship. Our marriage has been as perfect as possible.

We were blessed to live a year each in two different countries and visited others. Meeting persons of other cultures were life-changing events that brought us together even closer. We never tired of togetherness. Our special away-from-home activities included spending time at our vacation home in Anchor Bay, Mendocino County; tent camping in wonderful California state parks; and backpacking in wilderness areas in California, Nevada, and other states. These outings were always time to relax and get away from intensity of daily commitments.

Lifelong friends in the United States and foreign countries were special blessings who brought added dimensions to our marriage. Those who helped us celebrate our 50th, 60th and 62nd marriage anniversaries provided wonderful memories. For more than six decades, we have been blessed to share love given by power of the Holy Spirit that officially started on a 1952 October moonlit night at Coit Tower overlooking the City by the Bay, the Pearl of the Pacific.

The becoming of one flesh has, by the grace of God, taken us to the beginning of our 63rd year together. Carolyn has been one in a hundred million as wife and mother. Her strongest attributes have always been a positive outlook combined with a very high IQ. She provided a venue for me to become professionally successful as she did all the family business, shopping, and tending to the continual needs of three children. I could not have been more fortunate than to marry Carolyn Simon, as she became my best friend as well as a loving wife and example of grace to everyone she met, especially to me.

CHAPTER 16

Admission to Veterinary School

"Not all those who wander are lost."

– John Ronald Reuel Tolkien

The Boy With the Wounded Thumb had continually experienced anxiety after application to veterinary school in 1951. I would learn that June about my acceptance in or rejection from veterinary school. The long-awaited letter arrived June 7, 1951, from Registrar Howard B. Shonz; I had been accepted to begin a four year veterinary degree program. I had awaited this moment for 18 years, ever since Dr. R.F. Rasmussen saved my thumb on a drought-stricken Minnesota farm during the Great Depression. I immediately shared that moment of elation by telephone with Mom, who broke down in tears of gladness, then with Carolyn and several good friends, all extremely happy for me. I always will remember that moment of emotional high – the gift of opportunity to achieve my deep desire to be a veterinarian, and fulfillment of constant prayers asking for acceptance – thanks be to God.

Employment for three months at the MacDougal feedlot in Collinsville, California, 30 miles south of Dixon, a summer of 10-hour workdays, six days a week, gave me additional experience with animals before I began veterinary school in September 1951.

UNIVERSITY OF CALIFORNIA

OFFICE OF THE REGISTRAR
DAVIS, CALIFORNIA

June 7, 1951

Mr. Gordon Theilen
ASCA Store
Davis Campus

Dear Mr. Theilen:

The Committee on Admissions announces with
pleasure your acceptance to the School of
Veterinary Medicine, University of California,
Davis Campus for the fall semester 1951-52.

Please notify this office by June 20, 1951
if you are prepared to enter the course this
year.

Sincerely yours,

HOWARD B. SHONTZ
Registrar

HBS:rs

My letter of admission acceptance from UC Davis.

I was among 55 newly admitted classmates from various educational backgrounds. Upon completing three years of pre-vet courses I was admitted on my first application, while others had applied up to several times. Fifty-four of those admitted in our class graduated with a DVM degree. Malcom Brown developed Hodgkin's disease and died during the junior year. It was a scholastically outstanding class that led to wonderful lifelong friendships.

Class of 1955

William R. Bayliss

Lawrence J. Berry

Raymond M. Bloom

Howard E. Bond

Robert M. Bramman

Malcom Brown

Ralph R. Buon-Cristiani

Homer T. Caston

Griffith T. Clark

Denny G. Constanine

Ray R. Crookshanks

Jack A. Darling

Russell E. Douthit

John M. Eriksson

Jack Faivus

Fredrick S. Foote

Ted G. Garten

Henry C. Gregg

Keith L. Haydon

Joe R. Held

John T. Hollister

Arlen F. Kantor

Alex J. Kniazeff

Robert M. Lee

Louis P. Mack

Valentine J. Marasco

Donald E. Martinelli

Roy E. Mountain

James T. Murphy

Robert H. Nagle

Charles B. Nelson

Harry Oja

Robert D. Olsen

Olin Paul

Milburn W. Reed

Edward L. Roberts

Reynout Roland-Holst

William E. Rushworth

Mervyn B. Shenson

Edward M. Smith

Ralph A. Smith

Thomas N. Snortum

Gordon H. Theilen

Douglas J. Vance

William B. Wetmore

John Wheaton

Robert W. Wichmann

Jackson D. Wood

Robert L. Woolf

Ben York Jr.

John Young

Most classmates had interesting careers. Our 50th class reunion in June 2005 was an opportunity to see former classmates, some for the first time since graduation. Age had taken its toll; however, reunion enthusiasm existed for two days of seeing each other, with warm handshakes, and hugs from spouses as well as classmates. The 60th class reunion on October 2–5, 2015, brought together seven classmates. Togetherness was evident but not as enthusiastic as the reunion held 10 years earlier.

Freshman 1951

My first semester of veterinary school was almost a disaster as I was spending too much time with my wife-to-be and not enough time studying. I moved from West Hall along with Ed Nevin, my roommate, and thereafter we lived in the Beef Barn and ate meals in the cafeteria for farm laborers. Jim Pollock was the herdsman and we did morning and evening chores. I had sleeping quarters and a study desk that I reached by climbing a ladder hand over hand to the room above the other living rooms in the barn. These climbs to my room reminded me of my boyhood days catching pigeons by climbing a vertical ladder in a haymow to the hay carrier, then hand over hand swinging forward to reach the cupola, where I pulled myself in to reach and catch the birds.

Jim, Ed, and I would discuss philosophies in education, politics, and occasionally religion. Jim was a non practicing Christian who later became a husband and father involved in organized religion, a member of Davis Community Church. Ed was a non- practicing Jew but held onto Jewish values. As a dedicated Christian in the Lutheran denomination, I held onto devout views of God and his Word recorded in the Holy Bible, both the Old and New Testaments. I lived in the Beef Barn for about a year until Carolyn and I were married in 1953.

The beginning lectures and labs were almost totally dedicated to anatomy with Dr. Logan M. Julian as our professor. He had been a member of the Veterinary Science Department at UC Berkeley before transferring to Davis and the initiation of the Veterinary School. Dr. Julian was a taskmaster in getting student attention and meant for them to learn every bone, joint, muscle, and blood vessel in the bodies of various domesticated animals. The standard by which veterinary students learned anatomy was a wonderfully detailed textbook titled *The Anatomy of the Domestic Animals,* by Septimus Sisson and James Grossman, professors of anatomy at Ohio State University. Published by W. B. Saunders Company initially in 1938, this wonderful book contained

770 illustrations and was immensely detailed in animal species, particularly the horse and farm animals. Much less detail was given to anatomy of the dog and cat.

Most of the seniors were World War II military veterans who had missed most of their late teenage boyhood fun. Unfortunately for me, they had a voracious appetite for practicing pranks into their mid- to late 20s. Page 146 of the third edition of *The Anatomy of the Domestic Animals* described a horse scapula, the shoulder bone. Freshmen were forced by the senior classmates to wear around their necks a bone until they obtained signatures from all in the senior class at completion of the first semester. I choose the horse scapula and obtained signatures from all of the senior classmates before the end of the semester and thereafter I no longer needed to wear the large horse cadaver scapula bone.

To expand upon anatomic structure, Dr. Julian quizzed students on description of function and use of a certain joint or muscle. He had a pointer that was about three feet long and made from a dried stiff bull's penis. It looked somewhat like a wooden stick and a student might be prodded in the ribs with the bull's reproductive organ if he could not come up with the correct answer when orally quizzed in front of other students. It was a form of intimidation that no longer is used in professional education. There are weaknesses in modern educational progressive movements as depth for real thinking by an educator can no longer take place because satire needed in life is gone from teaching.

My classmates who were military veterans were accustomed to officers and non-commissioned officers giving orders with intimidating remarks and repeated use of the f-word. Some professors likewise commonly used satirical approaches in teaching, including aggressive gestures and insults. John Wheat, a surgeon specializing in large animals, was an expert in intimidation and aggressive teaching methods. If a student fell asleep in class, he forcefully threw a blackboard eraser at him. After being hit hard with an eraser, few students again fell asleep, even in the hour right after lunch, when he presented his lectures.

In the anatomy lab, anesthetized horses, cattle, sheep, and dogs were embalmed before death. An acrylic substance colored red for arteries and blue for veins was injected into the anesthetized animal to send the substance throughout the body. This allowed us in dissections to follow the blood vessels from the heart to the rest of the body. That was an excellent way for us to learn distribution of blood vessels and function.

Dr. Julian was a fast speaker, and taking notes during his lectures was difficult. Ray Bloom, a fellow student, took notes and typed them up for the rest of the class. Ray was an excellent student, with a photographic memory. He was top of the class in anatomy and continued as an excellent student throughout his educational career. The other outstanding students with excellent memories were Fred Foote, Don Martinelli, Bob Nagle, and Reynout Roland-Holst, who were Phi Beta Kappas. Five Phi Beta Kappas in one class was obviously special. The academic honor does not necessarily equate with original thinking, however, but rather with excellence in memory and studying for tests.

Those who made considerable contributions with originality to medical science and went beyond most fellow classmates and professors were Denny Constantine, Joe Held, Alex Kniazeff, Bob Olsen, and Robert Wichmann. Contributions from the Boy With the Wounded Thumb are recorded herein.

Dr. Denny Constantine, Ph.D., DVM, MPH, gained the rank of admiral in the Public Health Service. In 2007 he was awarded the School of Veterinary Medicine's Outstanding Alumnus Award in Research for being the first person in science to prove that bats can transmit rabies through air. He was a leader in all aspects of bat research and rabies. Denny should have been acknowledged at least nationally and perhaps elected to National Academy of Sciences. He used his mind and was a thinker, and had obtained a Ph.D. in microbiology before he gained a veterinary degree.

The tragedy of his education was flunking small-animal clinics in his senior year, taught by Dr. Lenton, a part-time surgeon who had come recently from England and was hired as a temporary instructor. One of the small-animal clinicians had suddenly moved elsewhere and an instructor was needed. Dr. Lenton remained one year, but while employed at UC Davis did great harm to my classmate by delaying his graduation and DVM degree.

Denny was required to take six weeks of clinics after graduation in order to gain a DVM. The person who flunked him went on to become a wine merchant. Wow, how certain persons can disrupt thinking and scientific advancement and be interested in selling wine rather than educating professional students while not realizing possibilities for original thinking and professional contributions.

The Communicable Disease Center (CDC, since renamed the Centers for Disease Control) in Atlanta already had hired Denny, as a veterinary student nationally known in rabies research, to conduct bat research. It was a great honor for me to nominate him for the outstanding UC Davis Alumnus Award. Denny was an exceptional individual who added greatly to science of biological interactions of viruses and animals, such as those seen with rabies infections. Interestingly, he was a student misfit in the view of many of his veterinary school professors but in scientific contributions he was a unique veterinarian, and internationally a leader in bat research and bat biology. He was responsible for establishment of state laws requiring vaccination of domestic dogs every three years for rabies prevention. In original contributions Denny was unique.

Dr. Joe Held, DVM, MPH, spent his entire career in the Public Health Service and was internationally recognized for research in global zoonotic diseases. He too became an admiral in the Public Health Service. He co-nominated Denny Constantine for the Outstanding Alumnus Award.

Dr. Alex Kniazeff, DVM, Ph.D., earned his doctoral degree while in veterinary school and concurrently employed by the National Naval Laboratory in Alameda, California. He did outstanding research in viruses and bacterial infections that caused chronic diseases. He was an immigrant from Manchuria of Russian heritage.

Dr. Robert Olsen, DVM, was a unique person who worked throughout his college career for various professors, helping conduct research projects. While in a small-animal practice in Hemet, California, Bob established a poultry practice, poultry lab, and poultry vaccines. This was all done in private practice on his own tine and expense. Bob continued to conduct a small-animal practice while doing poultry disease research. He exemplified original thinking as a professional, devout husband, and father, always showing a positive outlook in following a strong Christian faith.

Dr. Robert Wichmann, DVM, Ph.D., earned a Ph.D. in poultry diseases and did research in the poultry industry. He headed the private laboratory that Professor Bankowski established in Davis.

We were educated to become practicing veterinarians, and most classmates became large- and small-animal practitioners who were highly respected in their community of practice. I nearly flunked the anatomy course and at midterm had a D grade, but managed a semester C grade, which was sufficient to continue onto the second semester in school. I nearly missed my chance to fulfill my long-sought desire, for in those days, flunking only one class was grounds for expulsion. Even though I educationally wandered, I was not lost, and fully recovered to become a respected member of the veterinary profession.

Falling in love with Carolyn was a huge distraction from academic achievements in the fall of 1951. Serious courtships in most cases do not go hand in hand with being good students. The first semester taught me an enormous lesson, and I made a decisive change in class preparations. To improve upon our understanding of required information, Ralph Smith and I studied together each day. We tested each other on the subject material and from that point on I began to excel in all courses, especially in clinical medicine.

Faculty 1951–55

The first dean of the UC Davis School of Veterinary Medicine was Professor C.M. Haring, who had come from the Division of Veterinary Sciences at UC Berkeley. I have the work table that Dean Haring used in his office. Professor Schalm inherited it from Dean Haring, and in turn gave it to me. I used it as a work table collecting data for my early scientific experiments. When I retired in 2003, I learned that the wooden table was going to be discarded. To preserve it, I claimed ownership, and I still have it at my home office.

After Haring retired on July 1, 1948, his replacement as dean was Dr. George H. Hart, a UC Davis professor of Animal Science who had an M.D. degree in human Medicine. He was strict with junior colleagues and students. When Dean Hart retired, a more lenient person, Dr. Donald Jasper, Ph.D., DVM was selected as the third dean. I suspect the faculty wanted to rid themselves of authoritarian leadership. Dean Jasper became a good friend when I joined the faculty and was a considerate man. He had a strong family relationship and involvement in the Baptist Christian Church, supporting important causes such as the Gideons, who provide Christian Bibles internationally.

Construction of Haring Hall, the main veterinary medicine building at Davis, was completed on March 20, 1950, at a cost of $4.5 million. The 103,0000-square-foot building contained classrooms and laboratories. The entrance had a marble foyer that people in other departments on the Davis Campus referred to sarcastically as the "marble palace." Others on campus thought that veterinary students and faculty members were a bit more uppity than people in the other disciplines. In 1950, the Davis campus consisted only of the College of Agriculture, of which the School of Veterinary Medicine was a part. Veterinary schools at many other universities were independent administratively.

The first veterinary class at UC Davis enrolled in classes in the veterinary degree program in the fall of 1948, and graduated in 1952, one year after the Boy With the Wounded Thumb entered the veterinary degree program. The professors who taught students in 1951 were outstanding educators and immensely interested in teaching courses in veterinary medicine. We had an excellent education that gave the opportunity to excel. Several new disciplines were taught, including biochemistry, clinical pathology, hematology, and advances in clinical medicine.

Instructors for freshman and sophomores

Anatomy	L.M. Julian
Physiology	H.H. Cole /Jim Boda, Animal Science Department
Genetics	P.W. Gregory, Animal Science Department
Microbiology	D.G. McKercher, C.N. Stormont and Ernest Biberstein
Histology and pathology	D. R. Cordy, D.E. Jasper, Jack Moulton and Peter Kennedy
Biochemistry	Arthur Black
Pharmacology	S.A. Peoples and L.W. Holm
Poisonous plants	W.W. Robbins Botany Department
Parasitology	J. R. Douglas, Norman Baker

Instructors for juniors and seniors

Clinical pathology	O. W. Schalm, R.A. Bankowski, and D.E. Jasper
Reproduction	G.H. Hart, J. Traum, L. M Julian and J.W. Kendrick
Introductory medicine	J. F. Christiansen

Large-animal medicine	D.E. Jasper, Blaine McGowan, Ed Rhode
Small-animal medicine	R.M. Cello
Surgical anatomy	M.H. Schaffer, J. H. Woolsey Jr.
Large-animal surgery	R. F. Vetter, J.D. Wheat, Ed Rhode
Infectious diseases	J. A. Howarth
Poultry diseases	W.J. Mathey, Jr., D. V. Zander and L. Raggi
Public health	J. B. Enright and W.W. Sadler
Radiology	Ted Hague
Small-animal clinics	R.M. Cello, R.F. Vetter and T.J. Hague
Large-animal clinics	J.H. Woolsey Jr., J.D. Wheat, E.A. Rhode
Ambulatory clinic	J. D. Wheat, E.A. Rhode, J.W. Kendrick, Blaine McGowan, J. A. Howarth

Biochemistry was taught by Professor Art Black; physiology was taught by Professor Lou Holm, who later was terminated as a UC Davis professor for plagiarism. Professor Andy Peoples, M.D., taught pharmacology with an interesting flair for connecting medicine and veterinary medicine together as "one medicine," a theme of professional endeavors in the career of the Boy With the Wounded Thumb. Poultry medicine was interestingly taught by Professor Ray Bankowski, an expert in poultry diseases and inventor of an avian Newcastle virus vaccine.

Professor Cordy and young academicians Peter Kennedy and Jack Moulton taught veterinary pathology. Peter was an excellent teacher, especially in explaining detection of diseases during postmortem examinations of with myriad conditions and diseases. I was fond of his class and easily earned an A grade. Jack Moulton was a great influence by giving two lectures on tumor pathology. These lectures so interested me that I did extracurricular reading in the school library. Oncology became a subject of special interest for me. One piece of literature that caught my eye was a paper written by Dr. Ludwig Gross, a physician at the VA Hospital in the Bronx in New York City; in 1953 he published evidence of isolation of the first mammalian RNA virus that caused leukemia in AKR mice. The scientific community did not accept the discovery until publication of the repeated experiment in 1955 validated the existence of gross murine leukemia virus. Some years later I had the pleasure of meeting Dr. Gross and visiting his lab, and subsequently I received an autographed copy of this book *Tumor Viruses of Animals*.

Up to that time it was widely thought that cancer was a genetic disease even though avian leukosis (leukemia of chickens) was well accepted as an infectious disease. The working of the human mind comes into play in strange and mysterious ways. I have often been asked how I developed an interest in cancer research. I explain that it came as a challenge in my career; the veterinary medical profession needed to gain a better understanding and more knowledge about cancer. The discovery of the infectious nature of leukemia in cattle was a life-changing event for me; it was the coup d'état that cemented my emotional commitment to professional involvement in cancer research, which my book *One Medicine War on Cancer* explores in greater detail.

I wanted to be a veterinarian and contribute something special to the profession. I already was on the shoulders of great men, including Ludwig Gross, along with my professors who inspired me initially, and most importantly, Jack Mouton and Oscar Schalm. Professor Schalm, who developed the Department of Clinical Pathology, was one of the first veterinary hematologists. Veterinary clinical pathology was emerging as a special area in veterinary medicine in the early 1950s, and our class had the great opportunity to become the first veterinary students to be taught how to do complete blood studies and evaluate blood cell reactions to disease and inflammation.

Dr. Schalm was an expert on inflammation of the bovine mammary gland (mastitis). The udder of dairy cows was genetically selected for production of milk for human consumption. Mastitis was poorly understood until Dr. Schalm began to study its causes. Beef cattle very rarely developed mastitis, while dairy cattle were frequently afflicted, except on dairies where cows were milked by hand, not by milking machines. Dr. Schalm's research revealed that milking dairy cattle in poor sanitary conditions and improper use of milking machines were the major causes of mastitis. When cattle became infected with certain strains of bacteria, it spread from cow to cow through contaminated teat cups on the milking machines.

Dr. Schalm was my preveterinary curriculum advisor and told me that in order to get into veterinary school, I must take Analytical Chemistry and earn a B or higher grade. When I was an undergraduate, my grades were good, but created doubt about my ability to cut it in veterinary school. Chemistry 5 was a tough course in which many students failed or barely maintained a passing grade. It was not a requirement to get into veterinary school, but I enrolled upon Dr. Schalm's suggestion and received a B+ final grade. This let the admissions committee know that I had the ability to take difficult courses and academically achieve at a high level.

Dr. Schalm smoked cigars and was personable with students, who were required to give an oral term paper. My classmate Bill Whetmore (who after gradation became our class ambassador as liaison with the School of Veterinary Medicine) chose mastitis as the subject of his oral report, during which he repeatedly referred to cows' teats as "tits," before correcting himself – "I mean teats." This went on for several minutes until Professor Schalm finally said, "wait, Bill, I want to get you straight on the terminology of teat and tit." He went to the blackboard, wrote each word on it, and then said to Bill and the class "teats are on cows, and tits are on women." This brought the class of 54 men to laughter, and Bill Whetmore finished his report without referring to tits again. In the 50th reunion of our class, Bill accurately and colorfully recounted that incident. Such comments would not have been tolerated after the initiation of the feminist movement in the 1980s, since which time females constitute a substantial percentage of veterinary students. Huge societal changes occur in what is acceptable use of language over time.

My goal was to become a large-animal practitioner, like Dr. R. F. Rasmussen who had saved my thumb in 1933. Likewise, Dr. Seymour Roberts initially did large-animal work, and Dr. Bob Walker was an excellent large-animal practitioner. These men really shaped my interest in becoming a large-animal practicing veterinarian. In the summer of 1954, I worked for Dr. Stafford (DVM, Kansas State University) in the Marin County town of Novato, where I gained additional large-animal practice experience. I inseminated cows and assisted in surgery and, of course, cleaned kennels and did other needed odd jobs around the practice. I again found myself at nights being a babysitter, even though by now I was the father of my 10-month-old youngster, Kyle. I lived for the summer, however, at Stafford's facility, and Carolyn and Kyle lived in Davis, 75 miles distant.

Dr. Blaine McGowan was an inspirational clinician in ovine (sheep) medicine in the School of Veterinary Medicine's Ambulatory Clinic. He was a fantastic teacher and lecturer. Dr. John Kendrick was an exceptional teacher in large-animal reproduction, which became a special interest of mine during my first four years on the UC Davis faculty. Dr. Ed Rhode, a young clinician who came from Kansas State University was an articulate teacher and taught cardiology. Dr. John Wheat was an excellent equine surgeon, but I learned little from him because he wanted to be the only one who knew how to do certain surgeries, and would not show or teach others what he knew. He taught students only routine procedures, such as castrations and dehorning. He died in 2009 from Alzheimer's disease. Professor Bob Cello was an excellent lecturer and a dedicated small-animal specialist, a leader in new veterinary disciplines, and became among the first academic veterinary ophthalmologists at UC Davis.

Bob led the formation of specialties in the UC Davis School of Veterinary Medicine, which became the nation's first veterinary school to develop subspecialties. Bob was the first director of the newly created UC Davis Veterinary Teaching Hospital, which was the world's first academic veterinary hospital. Dean William (Bill) Pritchard DVM, Ph.D., spearheaded financial arrangements and vision that helped development of the specializations. In 1970, I became the director of the world's first established academic program specializing in veterinary cancer medicine. This opportunity was possible because of Dean Bill Pritchard's leadership and Dr. Bob Cello's original thinking, as *One Medicine War on Cancer* describes.

We had excellent professors and learned the latest in 1955 about Veterinary Medicine, believing there was no more to learn than what had been taught. Medical knowledge has burgeoned since, with new discoveries revealed almost daily nowadays. Veterinary scientists today must be prepared to dedicate themselves to continual learning. The way to become equipped to conduct viral oncology research and to develop the specialty of veterinary cancer medicine was through self-learning and innovation. As I entered veterinary practice following graduation, I immediately gained new knowledge that I had not found in textbooks or heard in the classroom.

The last semester of the senior year, a clinical practical examination took all day to complete. It encompassed knowledge from the entire clinical curriculum and all four years of education. The clinical practical exam was intended to prepare students for graduation and taking state board examinations. In that test, I ranked fourth, as a result of not doing well on one procedure. In clinics, students had the opportunity to think and assemble material learned during the first two years in diagnosing and treating animals that needed medical attention. At that point in my educational career, I recalled the words that Mildred Wiegers had written in a high school yearbook: "To the moron with the highest IQ in school." I doubt that the Boy With the Wounded Thumb had the highest IQ in the veterinary school class of 1955, but I had a great desire to discover new phenomena. I was not intimidated about trying new approaches, and sought answers to unexplained phenomena. "The mother of creativity is action with divine guidance" was a motto I used throughout my career.

In June 1955 I attained a goal – awarding of a doctor of veterinary medicine degree. I had longed to become a veterinarian since age 5, inspired by my hero, large-animal practitioner Dr. R.F. Rasmussen, who had obtained his DVM degree from Iowa State University College of Veterinary Medicine in 1931.

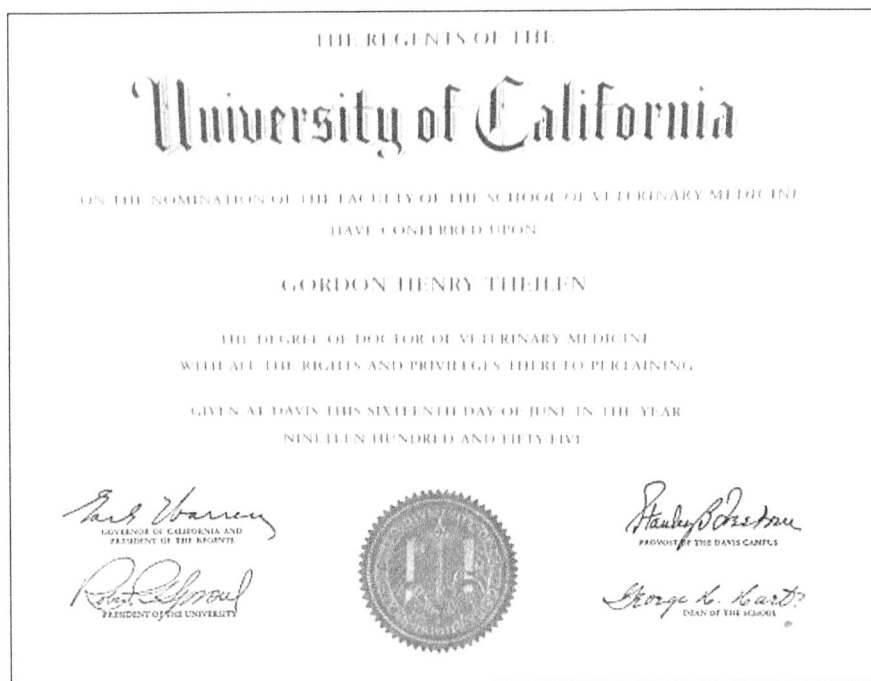

My DVM Diploma, awarded in June 1955. It was a steppingstone to fight the "One Medicine War on Cancer."

That veterinary degree meant that opportunities for me to think, teach, and develop new ways to add to the profession were now within the realm of possibility. I could guide and inspire students just as Dr. Seymour Roberts, DVM, of the Michigan State University College of Veterinary Medicine had motivated me when I was in high school ten years earlier. I derived my enthusiasm for making new discoveries from my associations with professors McKercher, Cordy, Moulton, Kennedy, Schalm, Howarth, McGowan, Cello, Rhode, Kendrick and others. Oscar Schalm and Jack Mouton probably were most inspirational of my DVM professorial educators.

I had chosen the opportunity to work following graduation for partners Drs. Dale Sales and George Puterbaugh, who owned a practice in Tillamook, Oregon, on the north side of town on the west side of U.S. Highway 101. Dr. Sales was an accomplished dairy practitioner. I took the Oregon State Boards in order to practice in Oregon; the state law indicated that during first six months after obtaining a DVM degree, a new veterinarian must work as an intern with an established Oregon licensed practitioner.

I was scheduled to begin employment with Drs. Sales and Puterbaugh in July 1955. However, a few weeks before my graduation, Carolyn became severely ill with an abdominal infection, first thought to be appendicitis. Exploratory surgery revealed that she was in early pregnancy, and had a fallopian tube infection with peritonitis. She lost the fetus and required several weeks to recover.

Several months before graduation, my classmate Dr. John Erickson had been offered a summer job at the UC Davis School of Veterinary Medicine as an ambulatory clinician. But because I had to stay in Davis during Carolyn's recovery, he agreed to do an internship in large-animal medicine at Kansas State and asked Dr. John Kendrick to hire me instead for the summer position through July and August. This arrangement led to a life-changing event and eventual lifelong employment at the UC Davis School of School of Veterinary Medicine, with enormous professional opportunities.

John Erickson was a learned classmate who studied to learn rather than studying for tests just to gain a good grade. He was a thinker and a true lover of facts with a laid-back personality that many classmates and professors did not really understand. He did a one-year internship in Kansas and came back to California in a dairy practice in Hemet. At an early age, only 15 years after graduation, he died from a massive stroke. The profession lost a learned and dedicated veterinarian, and I lost an unforgettable colleague.

The coincidence of John Erickson's good Samaritan gesture on my behalf gave me an opportunity to demonstrate my veterinary skills and educational acumen to Dr. Kendrick, my boss, and other clinical colleagues. While I attended the Midyear Veterinary Conference at the Veterinary School in February 1956, he offered me a position as a veterinary specialist as an ambulatory clinician starting in July 1956. As circumstances developed, I decided to take the offer after fulfilling my one-year Tillamook commitment. A year as a veterinary specialist led to becoming a veterinary educator and research worker in cancer medicine for the remaining 37½ years of my professional career.

CHAPTER 17

Ten months in Tillamook

"A dame that knows the ropes isn't likely to get tied up."
– Mae West

On a Friday evening in mid-August 1955, we left our 20 month-old-son, Kyle, in the care of Carolyn's parents as Carolyn, her brother, Phil, and I drove from Davis and headed for Tillamook, Oregon. We carried all of our household possessions in a borrowed farm truck that was less than roadworthy. Carolyn decided to ride on a couch in the bed of the truck. Our first stop was in Redding, California, for gas and a restroom break; Carolyn was extremely cold and uncomfortable. For the rest of the night she rode in the warm cab as we took turns driving. We arrived in Tillamook on Saturday afternoon, unloaded the household goods in our apartment, a single-story former barracks that had been used during World War II for military personnel who were assigned to coast guard duty 10 miles south of Tillamook at the U.S. Naval Air Station at which blimps were based. Surveillance blimps anchored at bases and hangars along the West Coast were used to search for Japanese submarines and war ships. Later in August, Carolyn, our son Kyle, and I drove to Tillamook in our new 1955 Plymouth sedan. Upon arrival, we set up our small apartment with groceries. I bathed Kyle by holding him with me in the stall shower. The apartment, a half mile from the veterinary clinic and a shopping center, had a wood-burning stove for warmth.

Tillamook, on an Oregon coastal plain 60 miles west of Portland, is famous for the dairy industry and special cheeses made in the cooperative cheese processing plant owned by dairymen. Tillamook in 1955 had 3,000 residents. The Wilson River, which cuts through the pasture land and rushes into the Pacific Ocean, drains nearby mountains and in rain deluges spills over its banks into the surrounding low pasture land. The average annual rainfall for this area is 88 inches, and between September 1955 and February 1956 the area recorded 108 inches of rain from storms that extended from British Columbia to central California.

East of the Tillamook Valley, the Northern Oregon Coast Range is heavily covered with evergreen trees, mostly hemlocks. The rain forest goes almost to the western edge of Portland. In 1933 a huge forest fire extended from the Columbia River 100 miles south and literally burned the entire forest. Some of the tall burned-out trees could still be seen in 1955. Tall snags of those beautiful Hemlock trees grew along U.S. 101, on which I drove to make farm calls. Off Highway 101 on county roads running between fields, bracken ferns grew like weeds. Cattle forced to forage on bracken developed depletion of blood platelets that caused anemia. Chronic ingestion of bracken fern led to carcinoma of the urinary bladder. Poison hemlock also abounded on the edges of the serene pastures in Tillamook Valley and into the nearby mountains. In 1806 the Lewis and Clark Expedition wintered north of Tillamook at the headwaters of the Columbia River. The group experienced a cold and wet winter, with difficulty keeping campfires lit. That wet winter of 1955–56 that I experienced gave me appreciation for the hardships that the members of the Lewis and Clark Expedition endured.

Tillamook Valley is bathed in the aroma of seashore with the fragrance of kelp and salty air. The valley and seashore resemble the landscape of the Channel Islands off the western coast of Bretagne, France. Dairyman settled here for good reasons, as they brought Channel Island cattle to this faraway land to enjoy cool summers and enjoyable lush grasses as found on the islands. Monks had genetically developed Channel Island cattle in the 1400s. Jersey and Guernsey cattle originated on the islands. Cattle were genetically selected for dairy from the 10th century and were never crossbred after the 16th century. They are among the smallest dairy cattle, and do better in pasture-type management than they do as large herds of dairy cattle reared with drylot methods in which they are not allowed to graze. The Channel Island breeds are genetically prone to develop low blood calcium levels when giving birth to a calf. Most develop milk fever and must have an immediate injection of calcium gluconate to survive. I treated hundreds of such cattle in a period of one year – the most prevalent reason for emergency calls, often at 4 a.m.

The pasture grasses of the Tillamook Valley are always green, as in Ireland, Scotland, the Channel Islands, and other areas of Great Britain and Northern Europe. Humidity is high with little dust. The pastoral scenes are overwhelmingly memorable. Jersey and Guernsey cattle grazed the succulent pasture grasses that produced good-quality milk high in butterfat, excellent for making Cheddar cheeses.

Lessons from a goat and a skunk

My first farm call in Tillamook was for examination of a goat that had not eaten for a week. It obviously had a severely impacted rumen (the first compartment of a goat's stomach, the large forestomach that collects fibrous matter in the first stage of digestion). While I had seen a few goats in my veterinary education, I had not worked on a goat farm. I diagnosed indigestion and prescribed castor oil to loosen impaction, and suggested offering the goat highly edible feed. On leaving, I repeated what I thought was wrong with the goat, and added "I really don't know much about goats." The goat subsequently died. Well, when the owner received the bill for $5, he refused to pay because the young vet did not really know much about goats. That taught me a lesson that I never forgot from that moment on – never say that I do not know anything about an animal or species that I am examining or about which I am making a diagnosis. In such situations from then on I told the client, "I don't know what is causing this problem, but I will try to find out." Never again was payment refused for professional work that I had done. If I made a mistake and realized the error, I immediately told the client about the mistake, even if it resulted in death. I never again was ostracized from a client's good graces.

One practice incident could be characterized as either hilarious or disastrous. A client, Ms. Brooks, had brought in a young kitten skunk to have the scent glands removed. She had named the skunk "Stinky." I was chosen to perform the skunk de-scenting operation. It had to be done outside, where the kitten would be given ether by inhalation, as I learned while working for

Dr. Roberts. The two scent glands are located near the exterior of the anus. I used small forceps to clamp closed each gland papillae to prevent escape of skunk scent during surgical removal, and then I carefully dissected the scent gland and sac from surrounding tissue. After the operation, Stinky became a house pet, exactly like a domesticated feline kitten. It would go in and out of open doors and always return to the house to sleep at night. Stinky used scratch boxes like cats. One day, Ms. Brooks noticed the skunk acting a bit strangely, and picked her up to take her outside. Well, it was not Stinky, but rather a wild male skunk that wanted to be with Stinky, who had come into season and attracted the wild male. At that moment, the male became alarmed by Ms. Brooks' approach, and sprayed in the house. She had to discard carpets, upholstered couches, and drapes. So it goes when selecting a skunk as a pet.

Originally, skunk scent was used to make fine French perfumes. It is obvious to many that skunk scent is a valuable product in giving upper-crust women an attractive lasting aroma. Isn't it interesting that in the wild, the scent is avoided with a passion, as Ms. Brooks experienced. Dogs often are curious especially in upland game hunting situations, and get skunked. The Boy With the Wounded Thumb experienced getting skunked at 6 years of age while living on the farm in Minnesota by following a skunk into a drainage culvert. I always remember the lasting smell from being skunked. Little did I know that 21 years later I would be involved in surgically removing scent glands from several skunk kittens in Tillamook, Oregon. These animals make good and interesting pets, but must also be neutered to prevent attraction of wild skunks.

Dairy cattle

During my ten months in Tillamook I began to learn practical medicine and gained knowledge about making quick diagnoses and treatment decisions in order to make the next call on schedule. This experience gave me appreciation of the need for professional efficiency, especially so for large-animal veterinary practitioners. Workdays were long, often extending hours beyond the normal eight-hour workday. Making calls throughout an area extending from 20 miles north of Tillamook to 50 miles south of the town entailed considerable driving time. The new Plymouth sedan I purchased in June 1955 had 75,000 miles on it 10 months later.

Initially, every call was a new and interesting veterinary experience. However, procedures often involved grueling labor. This was particularly true when correcting dystocias (problems in birthing) on cows often unable to get up from calving fatigue. That meant I had to lie on the level of the cow while trying to correct improper calf delivery posture. On one extremely interesting call, I examined a cow unable to deliver by extending my arm into the cow's uterus. At full arm's length I could feel the calf's intestines, liver, and other organs. This was a calf in which the internal organs had not closed over with skin and facia in fetal development, and the intestines and internal organs were still on the outside. It was a monster calf in appearance, with a poorly developed head and a body that was round rather than properly elongated. Medically this calf had ectopic (abnormally placed) chest and abdominal organs known medically as infantile imperfecta. This is a rather rare embryonic sequel following conception and fetal development.

Either a caesarean section or embryotomy must be done to deliver such a calf. I chose an embryotomy – cutting the calf in half with obstetric wire to enable delivery through the birth canal. Ectopic organs were clearly evident in the delivered halves. The owner, his wife, and children were extremely surprised to see such an anomalous birth. "Doc, what caused that to happen?" he asked. I replied that it was an anomaly that occurred early in the calf's development. "Beyond that, I don't know what the initial cause would have been," I said. That demonstrated to me how fortunate all newborns are to be perfectly developed and not like this anomalous monster.

I was involved in hundreds of bovine obstetric cases over the early years of my career, starting in Tillamook. The first obstetric experience of the Boy With the Wounded Thumb was as a 10-year-old assisting my Dad, who needed a small arm to correct birthing in a sow. After correction of the first piglet's position, the sow delivered several little piglets. On a call 20 miles south of Tillamook, delivery of a live calf took an hour, which gave me extensive arm muscle fatigue. I also needed a complete change of clothing because I was covered with blood and manure. Upon completion of that delivery, I phoned from a nearby gas station and country store to learn about new emergency calls. The next on line was another dystocia, and the only person at the farm was the farmer's wife, who I needed to assist me. The calf was dead and dry, adding to the difficulty of delivery. I need to take extra caution to avoid tearing the cow's fragile uterus, a condition resulting from a decaying dead calf. After lubricating the deceased calf with soapy warm water that the farmer's wife supplied, I could then reposition the dead calf for proper birthing posture. I wrapped the front legs of the calf with obstetric chains attached to a lariat rope anchored to a beam behind the cow, which was standing in a stanchion. I gained the mechanical advantage needed to pull the calf by using a "trucker's hitch" knot, which functions somewhat like a pulley. As the calf advanced through the cow's birth canal, the farmer's wife pushed down on the lariat. That brought the calf forward a little; then I added a new pull on the hitch, with the long end of the rope attached by a slip knot so it would maintain tension until the calf was guided free. I placed sulfa pills in the uterus to prevent infection. These veterinary procedures cannot be done under sterile conditions.

After each such procedure, I changed into clean coveralls and shirt. I disinfected my rubber boots on arrival and departure from every farm. After that call, guess what: the next call was another cow with difficulty in calving. This animal was unable to get up and was lying in liquid cow dung. I had to lie on my belly and correct the delivery and used the same technique as the cow before, but this time it was difficult to use the sliding cinch; most of the delivery was accomplished by brute force. At the end of this call, I was totally exhausted; fortunately, it was the end of the day's veterinary work. When I arrived home, I was so tired that Carolyn had to pull off my jeans and slip-on boots, and I immediately went to sleep on the living room couch, not interested in dinner. This is a synopsis of a day's work in Tillamook dairy practice, which occurs in other dairy practices every day.

A high percentage of calls involved familiar conditions such as low blood calcium at time of calving and need for immediate calcium injections; inflammation of the udders (mammary glands) with need for antibiotic injections into the affected teats; placenta retention after calving; indigestion from hay and concentrates; or imbalances leading to high ketones in the bloodstream and calfhood diarrhea and dysentery. Exceptional health maladies led to special remembrances.

There were myriad clinically challenging farms calls. I rarely attended to newborn calves because most were obviously healthy or would not survive birthing. At Mr. Achermann's farm, one newborn calf was gasping for air on every breath. Heartbeats were loud whirring sounds. The stethoscope sounds were consistent with persistent foramen ovale, which I suggested as a diagnosis. In such cases, the fetal opening between the two upper chambers of the heart (auricles) do not close normally before or at birth. Persistence of the opening causes improper heart function with insufficient oxygenation of the blood. The farmer asked, "Doc, what can be done with this calf?" I replied, "nothing." I called the senior partner in the practice, Dr. Dale Sayles, who said "let's put the calf down, and I will autopsy it to see what is wrong with it." He did not expect what he found: a hole in the calf's heart between the upper chambers. When Dale confirmed what I had diagnosed, Mr. Achermann from then on always asked for me first, and my practice reputation in Tillamook took a turn for higher regard. The news spread throughout the community, and I no longer was an unlearned upstart veterinarian just out of school.

In my senior year of veterinary school, a newborn calf gasping for air had been brought to the clinic. Dr. Ed Rhode, the clinician in charge, handed me a stethoscope and asked "Gordon, what do you hear?" I heard a loud whirring sound, but I did not know what was causing that abnormal heart sound. Dr. Rhode pointed out to me that in the upper chambers of the fetal heart, the opening between the chambers did not close at birth. What he taught me about persistent foramen ovale gave me the experience to correctly diagnose the condition of the calf on the Achermann farm. Thus, the Boy With the Wounded Thumb learned that a practitioner's reputation is based on making correct diagnoses.

Carolyn walked to shop for groceries almost every day, pushing Kyle in a stroller, because our refrigerator had a very small capacity. Carolyn looked much younger than her 22 years. On one shopping excursion to town after paying the bill, always in cash (because we had no credit cards in those days) the cashier handed food coupons to her and said, "Here, your mother will send you back for these if you don't bring them home." He did not realize that Carolyn was the woman of the household. She missed her California friends, but developed few friendships in Tillamook. She met the wife of the editor of the Tillamook newspaper and appreciated her helpful friendship. We had little social life due to my professional commitments seven days a week, other than occasionally going to outings at the homes of friends from the Lutheran church.

We drove to Portland where Carolyn consulted with a physician who specialized in infertility, which she had experienced since the emergency surgery in June. These visits to the city allowed us to have a day away from veterinary practice. On one visit, we had a wonderful dinner at Palaske's Hillvilla restaurant overlooking the Willamette River, a special time. We enjoyed good music by a piano player who performed "Stairway to the Stars," which reminded me of high school gatherings when my classmate Lucille Mallan played it on the piano. Unfortunately, such good times while living in Tillamook were far and few between because I worked an average of 12 hours a day, six days a week.

We had a friendly relationship with Dale and his wife, Vivian, while enjoying meals with good home-prepared food. I had a so-so relationship with the other partner, George Puterbaugh. He had a reserved personality that made having a good personal relationship difficult. When I was offered a position at UC Davis, the strange relationship I had with George partially influenced my decision to leave the Tillamook practice. Our lives changed as I began my wonderful career at UC Davis, and I thank the Lord for George Puterbaugh because if he had been an easy person to work with, we might have remained in Tillamook until retirement or death. Things don't happen by chance; one's life is directed by the Lord. George has been present at numerous class reunions, such as his 64th class anniversary, when we had warm reminiscent conversations about Tillamook. I knew George for four years before he graduated in 1952, the first Veterinary Class to finish at UC Davis. He was a running track star at UC Davis during his education.

During 1955 Carolyn's father, Ray, and her mom, Doreen, had moved elsewhere in Dixon, from Pitt School Road a couple of miles away to a Pedrick Road dairy farm owned by Elson Glide's sister, Mrs. Kendell. The Glide property, bordering the south bank of Putah Creek, was part of the original Glide estate established in the 1870s as a large area of land ownership. Putah Creek served as the dividing line between Yolo County to the north and Solano County south of the waterway. Ray and Doreen visited us in Tillamook in March 1956 and stayed a few days. As a dairyman, Ray was interested in dairy farming in Tillamook and enjoyed going on farm calls with me. Kyle often came along. Ray had indigestion problems and had a hard time sleeping while visiting us. Upon their return to Dixon in April 1956, he had a massive heart attack during afternoon milking, and was pronounced dead upon arrival at a doctor's office in Davis. His death intensified our strong desire to return to California to help Carolyn's mom. Doreen a few years later sold the diary business, and lived in Davis for two years. She purchased property north of Anchor Bay in Mendocino County, where she owned a gift shop. She married Ewell MacMillan fifteen years after Ray's death. Ewell and Doreen lived near Anchor Bay until health indicated they needed to live apart in assisted living.

In June, on my last call in Tillamook, I had to collect blood samples from a herd of dairy cattle in which brucellosis infection had occurred. Brucellosis is communicable to humans. State and federal law required such cattle herds to undergo collection of blood samples from all mature cattle at six-month intervals for two years, at which point the herd could be declared free of brucellosis. Each cow must be restrained with nose tongs while blood is drawn from the jugular vein. The owner of the herd told me that my blood collection technique did not disrupt his cattle. "As a blood sucker you are really outstanding," he told me. I took that as a compliment because cattle frequently are disrupted by veterinarians taking blood samples from the entire herd. Herd animals communicate with one another in a herd, so a veterinarian must exude a sense of calmness and confidence in order to avoid disturbing a barn full of cattle while collecting blood samples. Quiet approaches make entire herds of animals feel comfortable without triggering their instinct to flee. Some veterinarians have the ability to make animals feel relaxed, while others never become sufficiently aware of animal behavior, either of a large number of animals in a herd or individuals. The demeanor to suppress fear in animals is a gift given few people.

Return to California

We left for California at the end of June, pulling a U-Haul trailer packed with all of our possessions, and arrived in Dixon, California, two days later. Carolyn was happy to live for a few months with her mom, Doreen, affectionately known as Doey. Carolyn's brother, Phil, and his wife, Pat and their family lived in a second house on the ranch.

The farmhouses overlooked alfalfa fields to the south and east, and free-roaming areas for cattle were on the west side of the property. Pastures were divided into areas for calving heifers and cows for milk. Several newborn calf hutches were located east of the red milk barn. An unimproved private road connected the farm with the Elson Glide Ranch to the west. In 1956 Betty and Elson Glide built a new home that had a swimming pool. Doey took Kyle there, and that's where he learned to swim. As a youngster Doey lived on the island of Jersey off the coast of France and became an expert swimmer. Grandma Doey well cared for Kyle, and spoiled him as did his Theilen grandparents.

CHAPTER 18

Setting Roots in Davis

"Simplicity is the key to brilliance."
– Bruce Lee

We purchased a custom-built home in Davis at 882 Linden Lane in the University Farms subdivision, built on former farmland. Construction plans for the new home did not include insulation in the walls between rooms. Dr. Joe Ogawa, a friend from my UC Davis student years and now a neighbor, persuaded the developers to let us install insulation as the house was framed. Carolyn, seven months pregnant with our second son, John, did all of the insulation work. It was a hot September day, and the synthetic-wool insulation material produced irritation and itching as insulation wool floated through the air and landed on arms, body, and legs. This was the working relationship Carolyn and I developed soon after our marriage. Working and enjoying leisure time together was a formula that gracefully extended beyond our 63rd wedding anniversary.

At the time, I was on an all-day call doing veterinary work with sheep on a ranch owned by Harry Peterson several miles south of Dixon. Sheep work in the summer was done early in the morning to prevent the animals from overheating. Other calls pertaining to different farm-animal species followed unless we had to respond to a medical emergency, which took precedence.

156

Free time was most enjoyable while living on the Simon dairy farm. I happily treated cattle needing veterinary attention. On one occasion at the Simon Dairy, with students along, I was standing in front of a cow in the barn where stanchions faced each other, with a walkway between for manual feeding of concentrate feed. I was explaining the proper way to place nose tongs for restraining an animal while obtaining a blood sample when, without warning, the cow jerked her head straight up and the poll (top) of her skull hit me squarely on the base of my chin. The severe blow knocked me off my feet, lifted me off the floor, and slung me several feet into the opposite row of stanchions.

My jaws at the joints seemed fractured, and for weeks the simple act of chewing food was painful. I had a scar at the point of my chin for a long time. An upper-cut from Mike Tyson or Muhammad Ali could not have been stronger than this blow. The practice of veterinary medicine presents high risk for injuries and sometimes results in death. Some years after his graduation, one of my former students, Carlos Besio, was kicked in the stomach by a horse and bled to death from a ruptured spleen. Although I evaded severe injury, I have several scars as reminders of various injuries incurred while doing both large- and small-animal veterinary work. My hands suffered most; my right hand was injured so often it became permanently swollen.

Our second son, John, was born October 17, 1956. John was a large baby with a long body and a serene personality. Kyle had cried loudly and frequently during the first six weeks of his life, but John was the opposite. He required little attention, from just a few days after birth; he entertained himself by watching a slowly rotating ornament decorated with butterflies and small birds. He grew to be 6 feet 5 inches tall with a laid-back personality, and showed strong concern for all the people in his life.

On January 1, 1957, we moved into our new house on Linden Lane, which was shaped in a "U" with two entry points from West Eighth Street. We quickly developed strong-lasting friendships with neighbors. Most people who lived on this street were like extended family. Art and Trudy Black lived on the corner of Linden and Eighth. Art had been one of my professors in veterinary biochemistry, and became a supportive colleague. Bill and Betty Weir lived just north of the Blacks. They were parents of two adopted boys who were good kids, but not well disciplined. Bill also was one of my professors. He taught animal nutrition in the Department of Animal Science. Art and Phyllis Haig and their son, David, lived two houses removed from the Weirs to the north. David and our son John were good friends. To the north of the Haigs lived Jim and Margret Boda and their daughter, Wanda. Mrs. Boda was a kindergarten teacher for our two sons and other Linden Lane kids. Jim Boda was my physiology professor for a five-unit animal physiology course that I took as a pre-veterinary student. I received a "B," which was considered an excellent grade in his class; he awarded few A's, and most students received C's or lower.

In the next house north of the Bodas lived Jack and Mary Cohen, their two sons, Greg and Jim, and a daughter, Jill. The Theilen and Cohen families developed close neighborly friendship. Jack and I had what our children considered antagonistic arguments over politics. Despite our differences Jack and I remained close friends. Jack was politically a liberal and I conservative. He was transferred to Maryland following the closure of the radar station west of Davis where he worked as a civilian Army employee. His move left a void in my life. Jack and I remained in contact, talking occasionally on telephone. On a business trip to the National Institutes of Health in the 1980s, I visited with Jack, Mary, and Jill in their Frederick, Maryland home. Jack by then was suffering from advanced lymphoma and did not have long to live. We had an emotional last visit together. The conversation was open about Jack's imminent death. He spoke about dying and the fact that we probably would not see each other again. Jack was a strong Christian, and together we prayed for God's will to be fulfilled. The Boy With the Wounded Thumb departed that evening from the Cohen home with tears spilling down his cheeks.

The Cohens' next-door neighbors on Linden Lane had been the Les McNeil family. Mr. and Mrs. McNeil had a small business selling and installing flooring materials. Les was busy, yet usually had time to chat about local and national affairs. They had three children – two daughters and a son, David, who was a playmate of our sons Kyle and John and other children on the block. After Les died, David took over his father's business and has done several flooring jobs for us. We have been in touch with David for more than 50 years. Interestingly, his wife was a native of Sterling, Illinois, the place where both sets of my grandparents originated between the 1860s and 1880s. Coincidences never cease to exist.

Our next-door neighbors to the north were the Beecher Crampton family, and next to them lived the Johnson family. Mr. Johnson, who used a wheelchair, was a co-owner of a farm implements manufacturing company in Woodland, the town eight miles north of Davis. The company contracted with the university to develop a mechanical tomato-picking machine in conjunction with a project on campus to genetically develop a new variety of thick-skinned tomato that could withstand mechanical harvesting. The tomatoes were transferred to a conveyor belt for hand sorting and then dropped for collection into a trailer six feet deep. Filled trailers were driven to a cannery for processing and canning. Farm mechanization was reducing the need for hand laborers to harvest crops. Living in Davis next to an eminent agricultural university provided such opportunities to know and learn from people involved in such innovation. It was a pleasure to be employed at such a unique university.

I was part of a busy three-man university ambulatory veterinary practice team. Calls often began at 4 a.m. and continued until late at night. That hectic schedule explained why Carolyn did the insulation work on the new home. I simply was not available during our early years of home ownership for home-improvement projects. Carolyn took care of a multitude of household and child-rearing chores, and she was immensely efficient. She never held a negative attitude or complained.

Another family on our block, the Smiths, lived two doors north on the west side of Linden Lane. When they moved to Washington State, they gave us four steel lawn chairs with solid seats and backs. Fifty years after their move, we still have three chairs. They serve as constant reminders of those friendly roots we set down at 882 Linden Lane from 1956 to 1993.

Bob and Lynn Campbell lived with their children, Jim, Carla, and Greta, a few houses north of the Smiths on the outside curve of Linden Lane. A strong and lasting friendship grew between our families. Bob was an internationally known plant pathologist and an expert in viral diseases of lettuce. I visited Bob, Lynn, and family when they were on sabbatical in Cambridge, England, in the 1970s. Carla was a tiny baby at the time. Lynn enjoyed making rubbed impressions of bronze plates found in famous English cathedrals. The rubbings were exquisite, much like black and white paintings. Bob and Lynn relocated in 2011 to the University Retirement Community in Davis, where other retired friends of ours, including Trudy Black, the Sims, and Marge Ogawa, also moved.

Carolyn and Lynn walked for exercise every morning after the kids left for school. They became in many ways sisters. Bob's father was a veterinarian who practiced in rural Minnesota. When the veterinary school at the University of Minnesota was established in the 1950s, he became a large-animal clinician on the ambulatory clinic, as I did at UC Davis. Our closeness with the Campbell family probably was due in part to the fact that they were Minnesota natives, as I am. In older age Dr. Campbell developed a central nervous system condition that motivated them to move to Davis to escape the cold Minnesota winters and to be near Bob and Lynn. Bob later developed a similar malady, prompting the couple's move to the retirement center in 2011.

One morning five years after moving to Linden Lane, I went outside to get the morning newspaper and found our four-year-old pistachio tree lying on the ground. It had been cut three-quarters of the way through the trunk about two feet above the ground. When I returned indoors, I lamented about the vandalism and how badly the tree was damaged, and that it probably would die if not properly taped and restacked. Our daughter Ann, who was 3 years old at the time, said, "Dad, when I get to heaven, I will tell you how the tree lived and grew to be a big tree." What a wonderful remark from a child who then and always since has exhibited a spiritual awareness of God's existence in nature. Obviously, I was concerned that damage done to the tree would stunt or kill it. The tree survived and remains alive at more than 50 years of age. Pistachio trees are slow growers to begin with. The leaves of non-fruit-bearing pistachio trees turn wonderful shades of red and yellow in the fall in the Sacramento Valley, giving a hint of the brilliant color produced by the hardwood forests of New England. The color peak in the Sacramento Valley fittingly occurs around Thanksgiving.

Hal and Annette Parker and their five daughters lived at the curve of the Linden Lane "U," across the street from the Campbells just south of the entrance to West Davis Elementary School. Hal was a World War II veteran and graduated in 1952, the first class of the UC Davis veterinary school. He returned to UC Davis after a few years in practice, earned a Ph.D. in physiology, and become a faculty member of the veterinary school.

One of the Parkers' daughters, Judy, visited us in 1980, while I was on sabbatical at Justus Liebig University in Giessen, Germany. Judy was an exchange student in Germany and visited for a weekend. She came to Giessen by train and was so happy to see friendly faces that she ran to us and gave us a big hug. A young person living in another culture can feel alone. Judy needed to hear her native tongue spoken again and see people with friendly faces from home. Joining us at a nice meal with Judy were Dr. Joseph and Grace Seto and their teenage children, Steve and Susan, from Southern California. Dr. Seto was on sabbatical from UCLA, and was working in Giessen with Professor Rudy Roth in the microbiology department of the veterinary school at Justus Liebig University. Dr. Seto, a well-known microbiologist, was an expert in certain bacteria.

The three youngsters had a joyous evening sharing stories of living in Germany. Judy told how the German family with which she lived introduced her to a cuisine much different from what she had ever eaten. A favorite food of her host family was blood sausage, which Judy described with hilarious facial gestures and voice inflections. Her description elicited lots of laughter from those of us seated around the table. We have not seen Judy since shortly after our return to Davis in 1980, but have never forgotten her warm smile and that weekend stay with her in Germany.

Bill and Jewel Sims lived on the east side of Linden Lane. Bill was a faculty member in plant sciences. Dr. Joseph Ogawa, his wife, Marge, and their three children, Julie, Janis, and Martin, lived just south of the Sims home. Dr. Ogawa was a pomologist known for his dedicated work with fruit-tree farmers throughout California. Joe had been interned during World War II with his Japanese-American family. Marge also had been interned, sent from her home in Portland, Oregon, to a camp in Illinois. Joe and Marge purchased a vacation home that bordered ours on Fish Rock Road in Mendocino County in the 1980s. We shared visits while at the coast as well as in Davis. They were salt-of-the-earth kind of people. It was a sad day when Joe died before retirement from a heart attack, and I lost another wonderful friend. Such losses have increased during the eighth decade of my life.

John and Marylee Hardie lived next door to the Apple family. John worked for the chancellor in university relations and fundraising, and each morning drove past in a five-cylinder Mercedes diesel car that he kept in immaculate condition. Marylee and John and their two children were good friends. After John died in September 2011 from a chronic illness, Marylee continued to live on Linden Lane.

For 37 years 882 Linden Lane was our home, where we raised three children. We made many friends in Davis, Dixon, and the surrounding area, attended Davis Lutheran Church for the wonderful years we lived in Davis. These associations helped set down roots not in frost, but in deep, fertile ground. These roots nourished us just as the valley oak trees that thrive in this area. Buying rather than renting a home gave us a feeling of security and permanence.

Over time, though, many of the neighbors who had lived on Linden Lane in 1956 moved elsewhere, and relationships with the new neighbors who replaced them were not as close. Few of the original residents of Linden Lane still lived there by the beginning of the new millennium in 2001. However, Betty Weir, well into her 90s, still lived there in 2015. Memories of our wonderful Linden Lane neighbors bring back thoughts of the golden era of our marriage. Our children were born at Woodland Memorial Hospital, went through school in Davis, and graduated from Davis High School. Two were baptized, three confirmed and married at Davis Lutheran Church. Our life on Linden Lane and connections with the town and campus brought continuous joys to our lives.

CHAPTER 19

Clairvoyance of a Loved One's Impending Death

"To be, or not to be. That is the question."
– William Shakespeare

Clairvoyance regarding the impending death of loved ones has washed over me several times. The last time I saw my father, the finest man I ever knew, was in March 1965. I was doing a fellowship and sabbatical at the National Institutes of Health in Maryland and had returned to UC Davis on a business trip concerning expansion of a bovine leukemia research project. I stayed with my parents for a few days before returning to Maryland. On my last morning, Dad stayed home from work as I prepared to drive around 8 a.m. to San Francisco International Airport. It was a dreary, cold, overcast day. After the goodbyes, I pulled the rental car slowly from the curb and looked back to see Dad waving farewell. He had a forlorn, saddened look on his face, one of almost pleading, "I have something more to tell you.... Perhaps this is the last time we will see each other on Earth."

I had never before seen this expression or body language at any time during my years with him. A fresh image of his goodbye expression remains forever imprinted in my memory. It was a mere short month later that Dad died of a massive heart attack.

My last time saying goodbye with my mother was in 2006 after a visit with my sister, Blythe, and brother-in-law, Hugh, with whom my mother lived for several years. Carolyn and I had traveled to Alaska to visit Mom on Mother's Day. On the evening of our return, we said our goodbyes and Mom went to bed before we left. Blythe and Hugh were to take us to the airport for the fight home. I had forgotten something, went upstairs and stopped in Mother's bedroom doorway to see her one more time, even though she was asleep. The room was not lit, and I was extremely quiet so as not to awaken her. Mom sensed my presence, however, and said, "Gordon, come here and give me another kiss goodbye."

It was painfully obvious then that I would never again see my mother. She was a person who could not hear without hearing aids, yet she had the spiritual awareness to know of my presence in a dark room with no movement beyond the doorway. Mom had a phenomenal awareness of the last time she and I would meet on this Earth. This memory also left an imprint on me. Dad and Mom, as parents, saw me through many impressionable experiences growing up, from my first experiment sitting on a hen to see how she laid an egg, to how I nearly lost my right thumb to an ax, to having the thumb saved by a veterinarian, and my being pointed forever after in the direction of wanting to be a veterinarian.

The love of parents cannot be replaced by another person's love. I had exceptionally loving parents who allowed me to express my individuality to a degree beyond what is permitted for most kids. In essence, I was a thinking adult by age 14 similar to my grandfather Henry Schaller, who came to this country from Germany as a 15-year-old with two younger brothers to start a new life. I inherited the desire to succeed from the examples set by my parents, grandparents, and great-grandparents.

I had the same feelings of foreshadowing when I last visited Grandmother Meta Theilen in Le Mars, Iowa, on our trip as a family to Bethesda, Maryland, where I began a yearlong fellowship at the National Cancer Institute starting in 1964. I asked Grandma (affectionately referred to as "Ma," short for the German "Oma") if I could have the family clock that was always in her kitchen. I remembered it from visits as a small boy to my grandparents' home. She replied, "Gordon, I promised that clock to James (my cousin, James Nanaga)." But she added, "I have a another clock for you. It was my mother's clock." She was referring to my great grandmother Anke Collmann (pictured in Chapter 11).

At age 93, Ma still lived alone. She went upstairs and came back with Grandma Collmann's clock. It had been in my great-grandparents' home when they had homesteaded in western Iowa, not far from Sioux City. There had been encounters with so-called renegade Indians, but never any serious loss of livestock or property. This was about the time of Custer's battle at Little Big Horn in Montana. Ma had told me about her fear of Indians as a little girl. When we said goodbye to Ma Theilen on that August day in 1964, she too wore a look of sadness that we never again would see each other on Earth. She died in October 1964.

As we returned from Bethesda in 1965, we visited with relatives in Minnesota. Grandmother Amelia Schaller (Ma Schaller) was living in Luther Haven, a health care center in Montevideo. Carolyn and I and our children had a nice visit with Ma, and as we departed, Ma said, "Gordon, you know what I would like to have now more than anything else?"

"What?" I asked.

"A big family picnic," she replied.

As I walked away, it was clear I would never again see her on Earth. I've shed few tears in life, but the feeling of sadness I felt produced abundant tears that streamed down my cheeks. I did not want my kids to see me cry, and turned away from them. Ma Schaller was one of the most wonderful and important persons in my life. She was always there for me as youngster, radiating a sense of stability that I did not have from my mother as a youngster. Mom was a person often in the throes of depression, which left me feeling insecure. Ma Schaller had a wonderful personality, never complained, was always positive and loyal to her family and to her Savior, Jesus Christ. Her favorite hymn was "The Old Rugged Cross." She was not allowed to go to school after the second grade and was essentially illiterate, but mentally, she was a wise and capable person. She was one in a million, and everyone who knew her realized they had acquaintance with a special person who many did not know was self-taught.

Ma Schaller's mother had died while giving birth to her in Hamburg, Germany. Her father, Herr von Bergen, remarried and immigrated to Sterling, Illinois, in the early 1880s, when Ma was 2 years old. Her adopted mother was not kind, and took her out of school after first or second grade to work in a restaurant to help support the family. Ma as a little girl cleaned tables and carried the slop pail (a bucket used to collect all unwanted scraps) outside, where it could be dumped. She was a short woman, 4 feet, 8 inches tall; her growth probably was stunted from poor nutrition as a youngster.

When Ma lived in the home she and Pa had purchased in Maynard after selling the farm to their daughter and son-in-law, Fern and Harrold Sulflow, she remained busy. Pa Schaller was handicapped and needed a cane to walk. She took care of him until he died, after which she no longer could live alone. She then gave away various items, including the horsehide blanket Carolyn and I now keep at home on our living-room couch.

These impressions of impending death are spiritually related to the Lord and His Word. We were founded as a family in Christianity in Davis with continuous ties to God.

Davis Lutheran Church

We established our church home at Davis Lutheran Church (DLC) on Eighth and B streets in 1956 and continued membership until 2010. (By then we were living outside of Dixon, and we transferred to St. John Evangelical Church in Vacaville.) DLC members, family and friends contributed, along with faith in Jesus Christ, bedrock for Carolyn, our marriage, and raising our three children. Fellowship at DLC helped us become stronger Christians and enforced our knowledge of our Savior, which in turn gave us an improved way to provide a lending hand to others.

Some who have left spiritual impressions on our lives include four pastors: Norman Steffen, Paul Krueger, Dick Smith, and Jeff Irwin. Norman Steffen baptized our two youngest children and led us in prayer at the altar when son John was in a coma at the age of 18 months with western equine encephalomyelitis (sleeping sickness) and not expected to live. Norman began higher education at DePauw University in Greencastle, Indiana. There he met the love of his life and future wife, Kathryn "Kay" Pierce. After a year at DePauw, he transferred to St. John's Lutheran College in Winfield, Kansas, to begin pre-seminary training. He graduated in 1949 and continued his studies at Concordia Lutheran Seminary in St. Louis, Missouri. Kay and Norm married on December 22, 1951, in her hometown of Minneapolis. After completing his vicarage (analogous to an internship) in Bismarck, North Dakota, he graduated from the seminary in 1955.

Norman was the first called pastor of DLC church in 1955 upon the initiation of the newly organized Lutheran Church Missouri Synod (LCMS) congregation. He was well known in Davis, had many friends in the community and was an exceptionally outgoing man of the cloth. A member of the St. James Catholic Church in Davis once told me that Pastor Steffen was more his pastor than his own priest from the St. James Parish. Pastor Steffen was like a little Christ who always preached the gospel of Jesus and salvation through His grace. He lived what he taught. Young men and women in the congregation gave a youthful vitality to DLC. Pastor Steffen organized a fast-pitch softball church team that competed in the city league. The league included a team, sponsored by Wayne's Men's Shop, made up solely of UC Davis athletes who worked in Davis during the summer. Our church team and the Wayne's Men's Shop team led the summer league with substantial rivalry. This competition led us to become known in town as the "Fighting Lutherans."

The 'Fighting Lutherans'

The pitcher for the 'fighting Lutherans' summer league softball team was the best in the league, and we also had a good catcher: Pastor Norman Steffen, our excellent team captain. In one game, I hit a ground ball and was running it out when the first baseman of the Wayne's Men's Shop team, Tom Parker – a large tackle from the UC Davis football squad – blocked the base pad. I ran into him and down he went. He came up with fists swinging at me. I got in close to him so he could not hit me, but all of a sudden an opposing teammate hit me in the back and then tried to put his arms around me. Out of the blue, Dr. Inge, one of our teammates and a well-known collegiate wrestler from the University of Minnesota, put one hand on the person who had me temporarily pinned and, with one swoop, threw him to the ground.

That freed me, and I no longer was on the defensive. Instead, I went on the offensive as Parker came forward and threw a huge swing at me. I evaded it and hit him with a swing from my right fist that landed on his left jaw. He went down and got up for more. By now, Pastor Steffen was between us, and that stopped the fight. Parker did not want any more. We ended up winning the game and thereafter we were known as the "Fighting Lutherans." Many of the UC Davis athletes respected us as equal athletes and learned that Christians are not patsies when called upon to defend themselves. What most of the Wayne's

Men's Shop team did not know was that there were many World War II veterans on our church team who were well versed in self-defense, with or without a shooting weapon. The Boy With the Wounded Thumb had been well trained in self-defense while serving in the 82nd Airborne Division a few years earlier. However, the hit I sustained in my back from the fist of one of the opposing players resulted in a separated broken rib that Dr. Hage, our veterinary school radiologist, revealed in an X-ray image. I also peed blood for a couple of days.

I apologized the next day to Parker, who worked at the city pool for a summer job. He was wearing dark glasses and showed me a black-and-blue face and swollen blackened right eye. When these young college athletes attacked the Boy With the Wounded Thumb, they did not realize they confronted a former 82nd Division Airborne Trooper trained to take on enemy foes and never back down from challenges. Davis Lutheran became well known in the community, and the sanctuary hosted three services every Sunday for several years. It takes full participation in the community to be well recognized as a Christian congregation, even if one has to fight for it.

Paul Krueger, who succeeded Norman Steffen as pastor at DLC, confirmed our three children and helped us grow in faith. At the time, Carolyn and I were DLC youth activities directors. Carolyn went each summer for two weeks to Tahoe Tallac Campground and served as youth director with a combined group from a San Francisco congregation whose pastor was David Rohrer. David was the son of Pastor Otto Rohrer of Trinity Lutheran in Richmond, who confirmed the Boy With the Wounded Thumb and was instrumental in the Theilen family becoming residents of Richmond. David Rohrer and Paul Krueger were classmates at the LCMS seminary in St. Louis in the early 1960s.

As counselors, we would take DLC kids on a weeklong backpacking trip. We became well acquainted with the kids on these outings. We packed and hiked for 10 miles, set up camp, fished, prepared dinner, and by the light of a campfire discussed faith in the Lord Jesus Christ. We remember with considerable joy these outings and several of the youth – Carla Krueger, Andy Lange, and others – who took part. Joanne Moldenhauer was a youth counselor and well-known mathematics teacher at Davis High School who was inducted into the school's Hall of Fame. Another church counselor, Stan Pesis, become a minster and went to the LCMS seminary in St. Louis. Stan was Pastor for several years at St. John Lutheran Family in Carson City, Nevada.

Paul Krueger became influenced by developing progressive theology at the LCMS seminary in St. Louis. This philosophy led to a schism at the seminary. Several professors and seminarians left and formed a new seminary referred to as ELIM (Evangelical Lutheran Church in Mission). This in turn led to a schism within DLC and a split in the congregation. A majority stayed with the facility at Eighth and B Street in Davis, which and was an independent Lutheran congregation for the next year. The American Lutheran Church Synod agreed to accept DLC into membership. This occurred during Pastor Richard Smith's ministry at DLC. Pastor Smith retired after 25 years of ministry and baptized our two granddaughters, Jessica and Summer Yeo. During his ministry at DLC, the American Lutheran Church, American Lutheran Church in America and the newly formed ELIM synod joined to form the Evangelical Lutheran Church in America (ELCA).

Pastor Jeff Irwin became pastor at DLC in 2005. He confirmed our two granddaughters. He was a good preacher, however, it became more and more obvious during his ministry that the liberal movement that had begun in Paul Krueger's ministry, somewhat less obvious during Dick Smith's ministry and then was accentuated during Jeff Irwin's tenure, ELCA had become a liberal synod where many of the Biblical truths no longer were defined as important and necessary. ELCA's acceptance of abortion, divorce, and changes in other traditional family matters led to dumbing down of biblically given Judeo-Christian theological faith.

Most DLC members were extremely influential in our lives, expressing love for each other; departure to another more traditional congregation and leaving a brother-and-sister relationship was difficult for us. But it led to new Christian friends and miraculously to new congregational experiences.

CHAPTER 20

Our Three Children: Kyle, John, and Ann

"It's like déjà vu all over again."
– Yogi Berra

For Carolyn and me, the high-water mark of our lives was the rearing our children. Overall, guiding and nurturing these wonderful kids on a scale of ten we were seven or eight in efforts to lead them. Given the opportunity to guide them again or advise others about guiding children from early age, I would urge a more consistent traditional or conservative approach and more discussion on subjects of great importance to one's function as a Christian. Connections to sound education in Judeo-

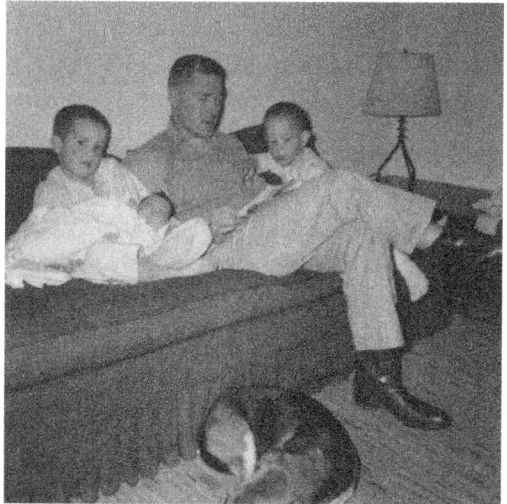

Gordon reading a fairy tale to Kyle at age 6, Ann at 1 month, and John at 3 years of age, with Lemmie the beagle dog, then 2 years old.

Christian ethics have slowly become agnostic or ignored worldwide. Other non-religious philosophies like socialism, with the state as the head of society, have become predominant worldwide, especially in Western cultures. There is less and less concern with living under God's law, maintaining a dominant belief in the 10 Commandments, unconditional love as found in Holy Scriptures, and holding onto strong ethics learned through religious education from family, church, and fellow moral human beings.

Carolyn and I tried to lead by example, and never criticized or contradicted actions that one of us had initiated with one or more of the kids. Thus, we were always together in child rearing, and if not in agreement discussed it between ourselves. I always remember Kyle telling the younger two when a correction was made, "Don't go to Mom if Dad had laid down the law, because Mom will always agree with his decision." Thus, Carolyn and I had no conflict in either the short-term or long-term raising of our children.

We held firmly to Judeo-Christian ethics and teaching. We faithfully attended Davis Lutheran Church, and the children were exposed to Christian ed-

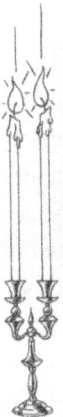

Peace on Earth

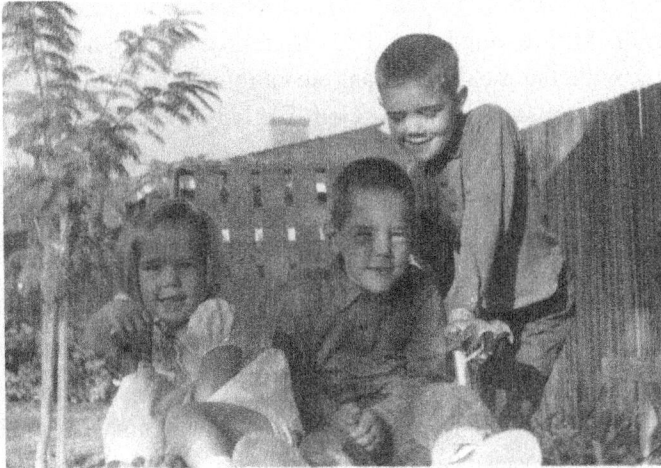

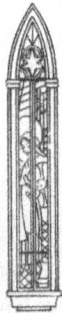

The Gordon Theilens

Christmas card showing Kyle, 8, John, 5 and Ann, 2, in 1961.

171

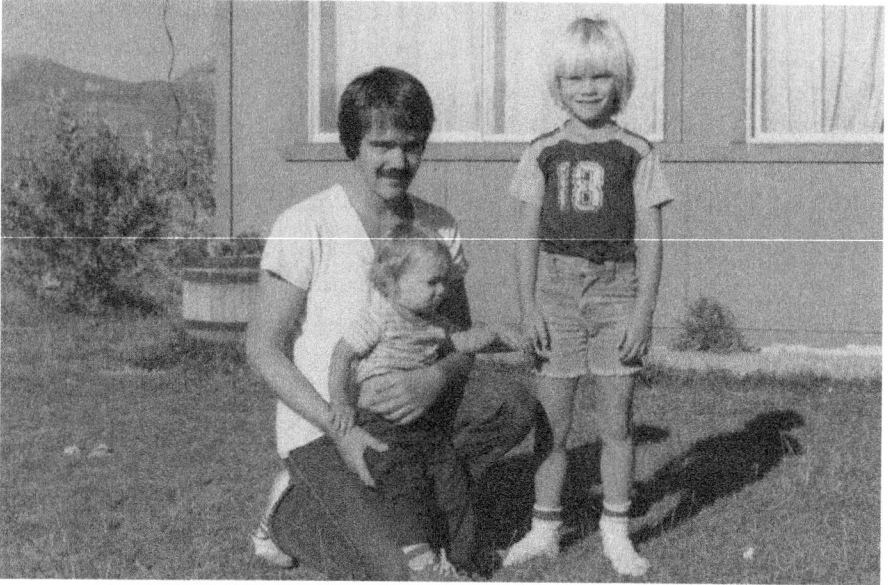

Kyle, Matt, and Joshua, 18 months old in 1982.

ucation there and at home. However, beyond always giving thanks to the Lord at mealtime, our lives were full of work, school activities, and other social needs. This left little time for daily sound Christian education at home. This is one aspect of child-rearing I would do differently. I would not rely so much on others to provide the most important educational ethic – that knowledge and wisdom comes from reverence for God. We led by example, but in the 1960s liberal peer pressure was overwhelmingly competitive to our teaching.

The early years went without a hitch, and the kids performed well in the early primary grades. However, Kyle, our oldest, started having problems with concentration and dedication to educational achievement. He continually was not up to grade level in most subjects, yet to us he always seemed bright and alert. He was noticeably intelligent, yet not an educational achiever. His difficulties in school may have been caused in part by too much pressure from us to do well. He was held back a year in the fourth grade; we thought doing so would help him catch up. The delay instead had the opposite effect, and his difficulties increased. We started becoming more lenient with the kids primarily due to Kyle's school problem and overall mental attitude. I believe that leniency led, unfortunately, to

Kyle becoming more and more secretive in what he was doing, so that by early high-school age, he was extremely rebellious.

This was epitomized during an outing to Bodega Bay with the church youth group. Kyle asked if he could take a friend who was not a member of the church, a request that we and the church counselor granted. At about midnight on the first night of the outing we received a call from one of the excellent counselors on the outing that Kyle and the friend had taken LSD and were having psychedelic experiences. This call was one of the lowest points in my life, because I had tried hard to correctly raise our children and guide them from doing foolish things. We as parents had a goal of teaching and exposing our offspring to become God-fearing citizens who contributed to society and added something to the next generation. In retrospect, however, we only skimmed the surface of ethical education and parental guidance.

I had been reared with a strong Judeo-Christian ethic, with my parents giving me a tremendous opportunity at an early age to live as a Christian and shun alcohol or drug abuse, which could lead to moral decay and deceitfulness. However, our society was changing rapidly while we were raising our children in the 1960s. The straw that broke the camel's back in moral ethics was use of LSD (lysergic acid diethylamide). This was synthesized from a fungus frequently found on wheat and rye bread that in medieval times caused large populations to go into an argumentative rage. Effects of LSD include thought disorders; temporary psychosis; delusions; body image changes; impaired depth, time, and space perceptions; terrifying thoughts and feelings; fear of loosing control; and despair.

Such persons as psychologist Timothy Leary, who had received his Ph.D. from UC Berkeley, and others advocated that purposefully dosing the world with LSD would be a righteous thing to do. Leary was arrested and imprisoned 29 times worldwide in the 1960s and 1970s, and President Nixon referred to him as the most dangerous man in the world. LSD was broadly used by the Beatles and other influential musicians, and by men of extreme corporate achievement such as Steve Jobs, co-founder of Apple. The Beatles and Steve Jobs were successful on the surface, but in reality led dysfunctional lives.

When I learned of Kyle's bad LSD trip, I cried and sobbed like a baby in total defeat, feeling that I was an unworthy father. For years thereafter his problems persisted as he rejected mainstream society and, unfortunately,

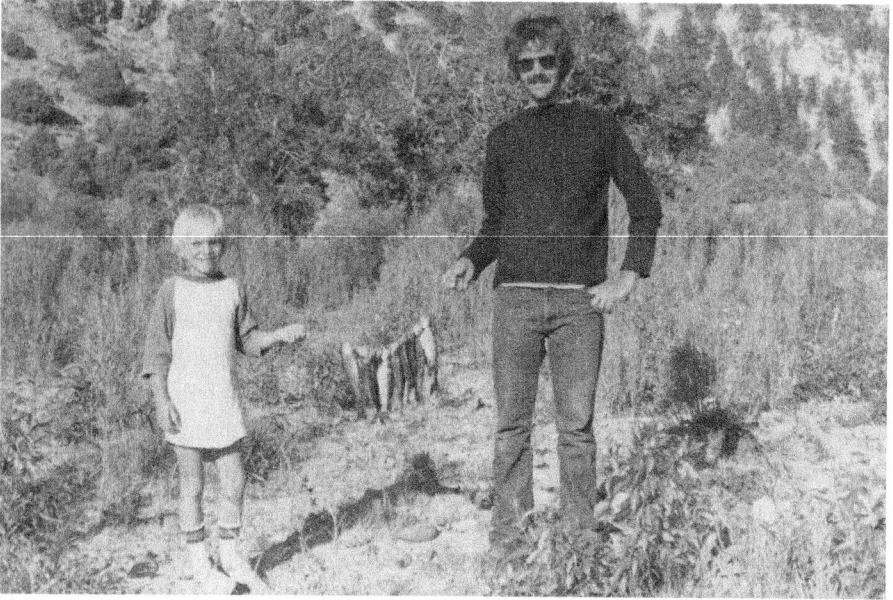

Kyle at age 29, with Matt, 7, holding a string of rainbow trout caught in Nevada.

becoming an abuser of alcohol, LSD, marijuana, and perhaps other drugs. The hippie movement of the 1960s, with its devaluing of moral standards, had more influence over our son Kyle than we as parents or the teachings of the Christian church were able to provide. We were so proud of Kyle when he was a little child and wanted only the best for him in his growing-up and adult life. He was destined to be good in high school sports and especially in baseball, but his scholastic achievement was not sufficient to allow the privilege of participating in school sports. He was never eagerly involved in any endeavor, and in retrospect I feel he was a constant drug abuser, but he had not showed full signs of it or alerted us to the fact.

For a long time after Kyle became an adult, he and I were unable to share friendly discussions. However, we developed more understanding of each other in later years and enjoyed most of all talking about gardening and sports. He avidly followed the 49ers and San Francisco Giants. Kyle and I settled on good terms and during the last years of his life he showed outstanding concerns for both his mother and me. He shared love for us, and that is what counts in the end in having and raising offspring.

Kyle died at 59 years of age on June 8, 2013, from chronic effects of substance abuse and starvation. One week before his death, Carolyn, Ann, and I visited him and his wife, Kris. We had a pleasant visit and, just before parting, held hands and in unison said the Lord's Prayer. I was dry-eyed and did not shed a tear because at that moment I saw him in God's presence.

Kyle's two sons, Matthew and Joshua, are good, responsible citizens, husbands, and parents. Matthew, the oldest, established a photography business and taught art part time at the University of Nevada, Reno, and a nearby junior college. He his wife, Tara, and their daughter, Zoe, have shown love for each other and the family, and we admire them as family members. Joshua lives near Seattle with his wife, Danna, and daughter, Jacqueline. Josh is a dedicated chef and enjoys life-endearing work of cooking and baking. One of the most enjoyable happenings in my life occurred at Trinity Free Lutheran Church in Dixon on May 10, 2015, when Jacquie and Zoe were baptized in the name of the Father, Son, and Holy Spirit. Our grandsons and family are close to us and show an enormous amount of love. They have happy, drug-free homes, and turned the tide on living a civil moral existence and revere a high moral code of ethics.

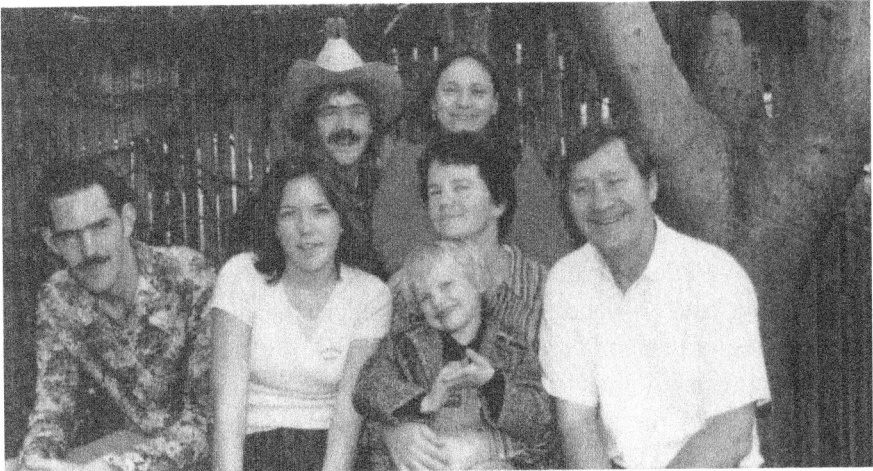

Our family in 1979, on the patio by a silk tree at our Linden Lane home in Davis, California. In the rear are Kyle 26, and Kris 27. In the front, left to right, are John, 23, Ann, 20, Carolyn, 48, Gordon, 51, and Matthew, 4 years old.]

John, our other son, never used drugs even though he grew up in the same era. He was a joy to see grow and mature. He was successful in school scholastics, achieved the rank of Eagle Scout, and is a dedicated child of God. He did show rebellion at times, mostly of a political nature. He left UC Davis while doing scholastically well at the end of his sophomore year to become involved in the labor union grape boycott. He intended to return to college but instead became more and more involved in union affairs, at the headquarters office.

John was appointed to the union's health care plan, and was administratively designated in charge. He traveled to recruit and take care of insurance matters in several areas of the United States.

On one occasion he called me for advice about an insured union member who was diagnosed with prostatic cancer that metastasized to the brain. The surgeon was going to do brain surgery. I advised a second opinion and arranged a visit to UCLA Cancer Clinic. The second opinion revealed no metastatic disease, and the man was treated for local prostatic cancer. All went well and he returned to work free of clinical signs of cancer.

The union leader had not approved consultation or medical costs at UCLA. John was fired for not following union rules for all matters first approved by the leader before any official action could be taken. This was obviously upsetting to John and us. We had always sent money and gifts to John because the union paid only for food and nothing for subsistence as practiced by some socialized labor unions.

As a sequel John became a policeman in Southern California. He married and raised two adopted children, Mercedes and Frank, and he and his wife gave birth to daughter, Katie. John in our opinion leaned heavily to the political left, with a negative affect on his life. While John worked on a tomato picking machine long hours of labor during the summer after his sophomore at UC Davis, he was led to embrace political socialism. He did hard labor encouraged by us to appreciate job advancement after college graduation. However, he was influenced by the political left ostensibly by a group that followed the philosophy of Saul Alinsky's book *Rules for Radicals*.

John was astute, and once he learned something he always retained the facts. When he was 10, I was going to spank him for something and he bowed his neck, stared at me, and silently said, "You aren't going to do that, are you?" That was the last time the kids received corporal punishments from us. Previously, it had always been done lightly and with concern for any physical injury. John has been financially irresponsible but has shown a lot of love in various ways. He has been an exceptional father and husband. Our granddaughter Katie bestowed the highest praise when she wrote in a note on her grandmother's 2012 Mother's Day card, "thank you for giving me the best Dad in the world." That note consummated success in raising a child and respect shown to a parent. It warmed our hearts as no other note from a grandchild has done.

Due to financial problems, John and his wife, Cristie, sold their home of 10 years and moved from Southern California to Virginia to live with their daughter, Mercedes. John continues to show love and concern for us and his family. He is considerate, with a deep understanding for a person's needs.

Our daughter, Ann, was an exceptionally conscientious person and gifted student who was outstanding in mathematics. Ann caused no problems in school, worked hard at Girl Scouts, and was protective of her brother John, who had suffered as an 18-month-old with western equine encephalomyelitis, a mosquito-borne virus that left him with physical disabilities. When he was in Cub Scouts, dexterity was of utmost importance in one game the troop played. As John ran to complete part of the race, Ann, then only 4 years old, jumped in to help him. She has shown this trait of helping people all her life.

Ann was industrious and started part-time work as a teenager by babysitting, later working at a Jack in the Box restaurant and doing other summer jobs to help pay her way through college. She worked as a waitress while in college. Ann majored in social welfare at California State University, Chico, and after graduation worked in Santa Cruz at detention centers for troubled children. This important work did not pay enough for subsistence, and she began working as a teller at the Bank of America in Santa Cruz. Later she worked at a bank in Davis and went to night school to obtain a second degree in accounting. This led her to a career with B of A, spanning more than 25 years. Ann always has shown love to us in many and various ways. Her love comes through at every Christmas and birthday celebration with most touching verses on cards for the occasion.

Ann has been a exceptionally good mother and wife. Our granddaughters Jessica and Summer have done well in school and shown strong interest in gaining college degrees. Our three children have been married and never divorced. They have guided their children to be responsible citizens eager to contribute to the community. In this respect, we feel we have succeeded in our endeavors to pass honor and respect in marriage to the next generation. We are pleased that God gave us three individuals who proved to be special in letting us know they loved us as parents and truly respected our efforts to provide opportunities for being good citizens in our society.

Family activities

Tent camping became a favorite summer vacation outing for our family. We took our first camping trip when Kyle was 5 and John was 2 years old. Blaine McGowan, a colleague of mine, and his wife Dorie lent us their tent, sleeping bags, and other camping gear, and we set off for Mount Lassen. Our plan was to camp in a section of Lassen National Park that was not covered with volcanic ash. I had not belonged to Boy Scouts, and this was my first campout with the exception of basic training in the Army at Fort Knox, Kentucky. We set up camp after dark in an area that we thought was covered in grass, but John and Kyle soon became covered with black volcanic dust. This camping trip, as dirty as it was, led to years of joyous family campouts in California state parks, and later to backpacking in various wildness areas in the western states. These were the golden years of our marriage, with memories of outings with the kids and time to spend long days together. In Davis, I was at work most days for 9 to 12 hours.

Through camping, the kids were introduced to fishing and nature in the out-of-doors. One memorable outing came in 1960, when we planned to camp with Ed and Lois Spafford and their three children at Burney Falls State Park in Northern California. The temperature that day was 114 degrees Fahrenheit in the Sacramento Valley. On our way to Redding our car overheated, and we had to flush the radiator before we could travel on. It was less warm at Burney Falls, at 3,500 feet elevation. The kids really enjoyed roasting marshmallows on sticks over the campfire. Susie Spafford is fondly remembered in photographs of her eating the gooey results.

Army Pass – golden trout

In 1967, Rick Morgan, a good friend and associate working on the bovine leukemia project, arranged a backpacking trip in the eastern Sierra Nevada. Participants included our family, vet-school colleague Bob Leighton, his son Robert, and another family. We drove from Davis to Lone Pine, stayed overnight in a motel, and the next morning drove to Bishop Pack Station at 7,000 feet. That section of the range rises precipitously to the crest.

Our goal was to cross Army Pass at 12,000 feet elevation and descend to 10,000 feet on the Western side, to set up camp there for several days. We had come the day before from Davis, elevation 35 feet, and less than 48 hours later were above 12,000 feet. We could look north and see Mount Whitney, highest peak in the continental United States at 14,505 feet. As we ascended, those in another family developed altitude sickness and were down for the next two days with severe headaches. We had three horses, and the kids took turns riding and walking. Carolyn and I were to share a horse, but I developed severe heel blisters from new boots and did most of the riding while Carolyn did most of the walking. Fishing was great in the Cottonwood Lakes area, where the golden trout were hungry and easy to lure.

In 1962 we experienced seeing the nation's highest peak, Mount McKinley (now called Denali, elevation 20,237 feet) in Alaska, while visiting my sister, Blythe, and her husband, Dick Stenmark, and their 2-month-old daughter Kirsten. Like Mount Fuji (Fujiyama) in Japan and Mount Shasta in Northern California, Mount McKinley is a prominent peak that stands somewhat by itself in the Alaska Range, while the mountains we ascended in the Sierra all blended together. The Boy With the Wounded Thumb ascended to the 10,000-foot level of 12,389-foot Fujiyama in 1966. It has been the object of pilgrimage for centuries and plays a large part in Japanese culture. While there was not that cultural sense in crossing Army Pass at 12,000 feet, the challenge and effort involved crossing from one side of a mountain range to the other gave us a memorable thrill.

During that 1962 visit with Blythe and Dick, he took me on a 24-hour hiking trip during which we locked ice axes together to establish balance as we crossed raging streams. We crossed a pass at an elevation of 12,000 feet where we saw arctic terns that migrated from Australia, covering yearly a 7,000-mile course. This hike was extremely amazing. We saw grizzly bears, Dall sheep, a herd of several thousand migrating caribou, and many wonderful birds. I was exhausted upon return to Wonder Lake Ranger Station, 80 miles from national park headquarters. Blythe and Dick lived at Wonder Lake for the summer months.

Mountains and the out-of-doors were our family's main source of vacation pleasures. These excursions taught us to appreciate the wonders of nature and God's creatures and creations. Carolyn and I often recount these special moments in wilderness areas as some of the best times in our 63-and-counting married years.

Backpacking

As our children got older, we began backpacking, mostly in Northern California. The Trinity Alps in Trinity County and Marble Mountains in Siskiyou County were favorites. We often were out for a week with scouts or a church youth group, and packed an average of 10 miles a day, sometimes as much as 15 or more miles in a day. Some of the hiking challenges we faced are worthy of mention. On a wonderful outing in the Marble Mountains, Charles Judson, a University friend, and I were leaders of Explorer Scouts doing trail maintenance. Marilyn Judson and Carolyn went along with the Judsons' daughter and our daughter, Ann.

The scouts left base camp and worked along the trail for two days. On the way back, we descended 1,000 feet to a mountain lake to fish. John caught a huge trout, and became snagged in a submerged tree. I took off my clothes, dove about 10 feet down, captured the snagged fish and brought it to the

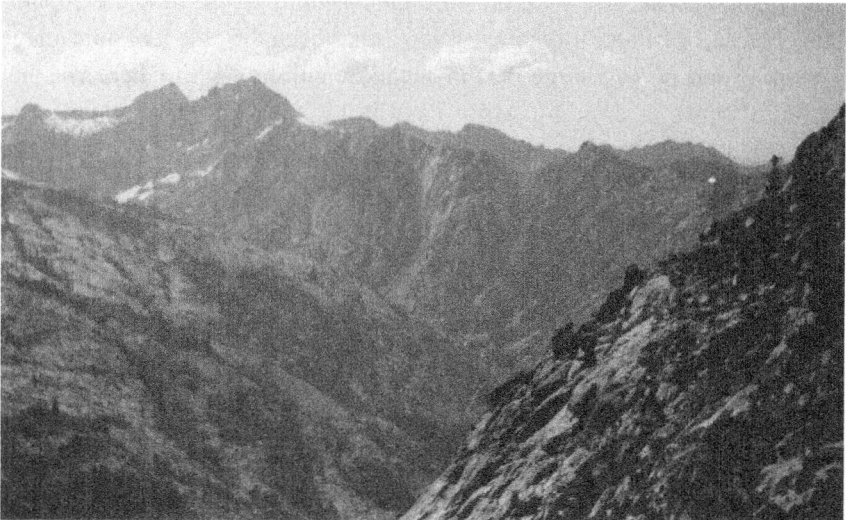

This 1971 scene in California's Trinity Alps shows typical backpacking terrain.

surface. The water was icy cold. After redressing, the Boy With the Wounded Thumb resumed fishing. Charles and the scouts began the trek up the mountain to the ridge trail to go 10 miles to the base camp. I remained and fished in the serenity of the infrequently visited lake, listened to various sounds, and saw an osprey swoop down and catch a fish, taking off flying with the fish held head-first between its talons. This pristine wilderness remains as a wonderful and lasting memory of how the West and the world once looked. Being there, I recalled descriptions I had read years before in Irving Stone's *Men to Match My Mountains,* a 1956 novel about the opening of the Far West.

While we were fishing at the lake, I heard the wind make eerie sounds like a loud wooing from a large voice. This, after all, was the land of Bigfoot, the mythical hominid-like creature some believe still inhabits these parts. Was I listening to Bigfoot? After ascending the trail to the mountain's crest, I looked westward as the sun was setting and fog was coming in from the Pacific about 50 miles away, and wondered if I would ever see this wonderful wilderness again. This was 1971, when I was 43 years old and in my prime, and I never again saw it from a backpacking perspective. The Boy With the Wounded Thumb began to realize one stage of my life was coming to an end. For the next four-plus decades, I have often asked in silence, "Lord, will I ever see this place again or experience this happening?" Frequently I rely on memories, as I often read a plaque on our bedroom wall that reads: "God gave us memories so we could smell flowers in the winter."

Nevada

We enjoyed our outings with the Breens from Reno, who I first met while treating one of Fran Breen's dogs, "Red," for an oral neoplasm. Red was responsible for two large grants from the Max C. Fleischmann Foundation. One was to study leukemia in animals as a model for a collaborative study of human leukemia at the UC Davis School of Medicine. A bit later came a $1 million grant to establish the Center for Comparative Cancer Medicine, which evolved after my retirement in 1993 to the Center For Companion Animal Health.

We packed into the Jarbidge Wilderness area in northeastern Nevada, near the corner of Utah and Idaho. This was one of the few backcountry trips taken where cars were left at a high point. The packing party descended into the Jarbidge River basin. As we walked through aspen groves, we saw carvings on tree trunks made by the Basque sheepherders who had migrated here years before. Fishing and camping camaraderie was outstanding.

A few years later we took a memorable trip to the Ruby Mountains, which stand as a range by themselves, rising to 12,000 feet. We stayed the first night in Elko, Nevada, and accessed the Rubys from the northeast side, not far from Lamoille. The party this time consisted of Fran and Ellie Breen, Richmond Breen, Carolyn and me. We packed to the top of the Rubys and then down into a basin and set up camp about 15 miles from the cars. We fished and explored the area. The mountainsides were sagebrush covered, and at higher elevations, consisted mostly of lava rocks dotted by a few trees.

A few days later, we decided to go to the south end of the Rubys. Richmond and Ellie packed across the mountaintops, while the rest of us walked back 15 miles to the cars and drove 30 miles around the base of the mountains, left the cars, and packed another 15 miles up the summit on the same day. We walked with packs 30 miles in one day. The next day, while we were camping near the summit, a vicious wind came up with torrential rain. We descended to the cars, and rain poured down hard all the way. A shallow creek we had crossed hiking up was raging with water two feet deep in a flash flood.

Totally soaked after going 45 miles in less than two days, we were greeted by a local farmer. He invited us in for coffee spiked with brandy, which helped take away the hypothermia that had set in. Carolyn and I left for California and drove to a rundown motel in Winnemucca. We were so tired we didn't care that it was a flea trap. The various mountain ranges in Nevada are extremely interesting and beautiful. Nevada is one of the least understood out-of-doors wonderlands in the world. The high plateau desert consumes one's attention. Few people explore the Ruby or Jarbidge areas. Interestingly, Nevada's watersheds are land-locked, and no water drains beyond its borders.

Uintas: Near disaster

Carolyn, Ann, Dee Dee Blaylock and I drove to Denver for the American Veterinary Medicine Association convention in July 1974. Afterward, we went to Utah and started in the late afternoon to backpack into the High Uintas Wilderness in the northeastern part of the state. Rain set in after five miles on the trail, and our sleeping bags were soaking wet. Starting a fire to cook the evening meal was difficult.

The next morning dawned with full sunshine, and we packed over a 12,000-foot pass. In early afternoon, clouds started forming again. It was obvious that an electrical storm was brewing. We stopped at treeline at 10,000 feet in a nice meadow, and the girls set up a tube tent between two trees. After we got our tent set up and the girls were settled in, the storm hit. Lightning strikes were occurring all around us. Many hit nearby and the ground sizzled with electricity. After two hours of unbelievably strong wind, hail, and snow, the storm abated, leaving everything around us wet and cold. Hailstones remained on the ground, creating a scene reminiscent of wintertime.

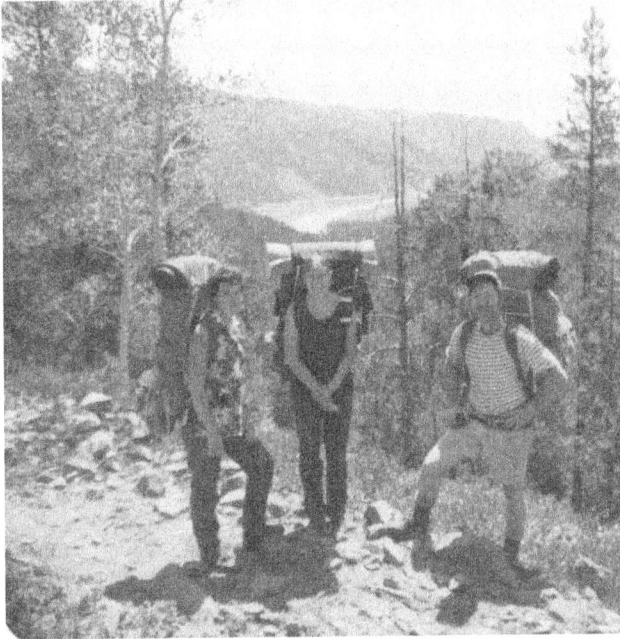

Backpacking in Uinta Mountains, Utah, in 1974. Carolyn carried a 40-pound pack, Dee Dee Blaylock hiked with a 30-pound pack, and Gordon lugged a 50-pound pack on a trail to a pass at 12,000 feet in elevation. Ann took this photo of Carolyn, Dee Dee, and me at our campsite at an elevation of 6,000 feet in the early morning. We were preparing to pack on an ascent through a 12,000-foot pass in the High Uintas Wilderness before descending to tree line at 10,000 feet.

After getting a one-burner stove going, we had hot soup at 9 p.m. and went to bed. Our bags were again wet, but we were tired and therefore able to sleep. All of us awoke early in the morning, and packed out to the starting point. Thus in two days we traveled 35 miles, all at high altitude. This was the most taxing and near-death experience of our backpacking career. After this packing The Boy With the Wounded Thumb stayed in Nevada and California, never again to experience a storm with life-threatening lightning close by.

CHAPTER 21

Animals and Plants in the Out-of-Doors

"God gave us memory so we might have roses in December."
– James Matthew Barrie

Nature's wonders

A special spin-off from camping and backpacking was the opportunity to feel and see the wonders of animals and plants God provided in nature. Trees always were inspirational to me, and from an early age I felt compelled to climb them. Medium-size ash, cottonwood, alder, and birch trees, along with evergreens of the fir family, were cultivated in groves around farms in Minnesota. These trees served as windbreaks on the north and west sides of farm buildings.

Wind in winter would bring an eerie whirring of sounds, almost Halloween ghost-like, that made nature seem scary and overpowering. Then, in spring, when the first beautiful light-green leaves appeared like a hazy hue over the small forest, there was joy. The sighting of the first robin, meadowlark, or blackbird migrating north made it seem as though a new planet occurred out of bleakness of winter.

Climbing trees to find nests and observe egg colors after the birds nested was a favorite pastime of mine. Robin eggs were wonderfully light blue. It was important to avoid touching the nest because nesting birds would not return in the presence of human scent. In 10-14 days, the eggs would hatch fuzzy new chicks that would spend four weeks in the nest before fledging and learning to fly. They still needed care from the parents for a few more days or a week after leaving the nest.

The technique I used in climbing trees was pulling my body upward with arms holding on to limbs to prevent falling; I wrapped my legs around the trunk of the tree until I reached the lower branches, which served as footholds enabling me to go farther up the tree. From there, it was a matter of pulling upward to the next branch and testing each new branch to be sure it would not break off, posing risk of an injurious fall. Climbing trees was a personal test to prove that fear of heights could be overcome. Life is full of ups and downs, and climbing up and down trees prepared me in a way for the ups and downs of professional life.

It is easy to be emotionally attracted to California's valley oak trees, the predominant species in the Sacramento and San Joaquin valleys until the advent of widespread agriculture in the 1850s. Mature valley oaks have an extensive limb span. Their leaves give off a natural herbicide, resulting in weed and brush control beneath them. The majestic oak tree; trees generally are stressed in 1913 Joyce Kilmer poem "Trees."

I think that I shall never see
A poem as lovely as a tree.

A tree whose hungry mouth is prest
Against the earth's sweet flowering breast;

A tree that looks at God all day
And lifts her leafy arms to pray;

A tree that may in summer wear
A nest of robins in her hair;

Upon whose bosom snow has lain
Who intimately lives with rain.

Poems are made by fools like me
But only God can make a tree.

[Public domain]

Kilmer was born Alfred Joyce Kilmer in 1886 and died fighting with the famous 69th Infantry Regiment in World War I's second battle of the Marne in 1918 (immortalized in the 1940 motion picture *The Fighting 69th* starring James Cagney, with actor Jeffrey Lynn portraying Joyce Kilmer. He was married and had five children when he was killed in France at the age of 31.

Going Over the Top, another movie dramatizing battles in France, depicted Sergeant Alvin York, who singlehandedly killed 28 German soldiers, and with the remnants of his squad captured 132 Germans and silenced their machine-gun nests. He was awarded the Congressional Medal of Honor. He was in the 82nd Division in the 328th Infantry. My uncle, Dad's brother Ben, fought in France with the 82nd Infantry Division. This division became the first Airborne Division in World War II and continues to exist into the 21st century. I was member of the 82nd Airborne Division in 1947–48.

Birds

As a family we identified birds. None was of greater interest than the Arctic terns I observed in the Alaska Range in 1962. On our ranch in Dixon, California, we routinely observe several game bird species, in a wildlife refuge on three acres of land with a manmade lake in the middle. We frequently hear and see pheasants, Canada geese, mallard ducks, California quail, and wild turkeys, along with crows (some of which act like pets), yellow-billed magpies, brush blue jays and mockingbirds, which have a beautiful song in spring and summer but are quiet the rest of the year.

From November though March each year, black-hooded night herons use our weeping willow trees as a rookery. At evening, when darkness begins to overtake the light, these birds take off one by one, returning before daybreak. When they leave for the evening, they emit a "quack-quack" sound, not like a duck, but one of their own. I call out to them and they call back as they fly off for an evening foraging. Their diet consists of crayfish and other species of aquatic life. When I go under the trees or near the roost, they don't scare. However, when unfamiliar persons are present, they scare and fly off. It is interesting that they are confident with me, recognize and have no fear of my presence.

This is just one example of wild animals becoming confident in the presence of humans who have not molested them. I often think of St. Francis of Assisi, who apparently attracted wild animals as if they were domesticated. According to legend, he went into the mountains from Assisi and confronted a wild, vicious wolf. The wolf listened to St. Francis's soft voice and lay down at his feet. St. Francis obviously was able to "read" animals and had special powers to attract them.

Francis lived a primitive life, was not ordained into the priesthood, and was a strong follower of Jesus (Matthew 10:9). He eventually was recognized by the Roman Catholic Church, and established the Franciscan Order and the Order of St. Clare (for nuns); he was recognized on his festival day, October 3, as the patron saint of animals. St. Francis wrote a beautiful prayer that fully expresses how he acknowledged the Christian doctrine and love for all of God's creatures.

The Prayer of Saint Francis

Lord, make me an instrument of your peace.
Where there is hatred, let me sow love;
Where is injury, pardon;
Where there is doubt, faith;
Where there is despair, hope;
Where there is darkness, light;
Where there is sadness, joy.
Lord, grant that I may not so much seek to be consoled as to console;
To be understood as to understand;
To be loved as to love;
For it is in giving that we receive;
It is in pardoning that we are pardoned;
It is in dying that we are born again to eternal life.

In reflection of this prayer, an animal lover can feel peace, love, pardon, understanding, joy, and consolation from association with animals, whether large mammals, birds, reptiles, insects, bees, or the insect of peace, the butterfly.

Some Christians believe animals do not have souls. The Holy Bible does not indicate whether they do or not, or if they will reside in heaven along with those humans saved for eternal life. Yet there is no doubt that the Lord God made them all, large and small. Veterinarians are charged with caring for all creatures in need of medical help. In the world of animals, the Boy With the Wounded Thumb committed a life of professional endeavor to add new knowledge to benefit animals and humans, "one medicine" war on cancer.

Dawn chorus

One of the most interesting aspects of the world of birds is the "dawn chorus" displayed each summer morning at dawn in England. I had the God-given pleasure to experience and hear the dawn chorus the entire summer of 1973 while on sabbatical at the Royal Marsden Hospital in Sutton, Surrey, south of London. In the mornings, thousands of songbirds sing an hour before dawn. Suddenly, after a loud crescendo, a quiet broken only by individual chirping set in. The next morning brought a return to the phenomenon that has occurred for thousands and thousands of years.

At moments like these the cathedral of life takes on a closer presence to God, maker of heaven and Earth and all that is in it. *"Let there be light, and there was light separated from darkness."* The dawn chorus begins in the hour that light brings deliverance from the darkness of night.

I first heard the call of a cuckoo bird when I was in England. It sounded like a playback from a cuckoo clock. The cuckoo bird lays its eggs in the nest of another species and allows the unsuspecting mother to raise its young along with her own. Yet the cuckoo mates with its own kind again, and the life cycle goes on with modified perpetuation of the species. Some people have adopted similar practices, but for the most part, whether avian, mammal, or other families of animals, the parent or parents are fiercely loyal to raising the newly hatched or born until they can fend on their own. The cuckoo is an exception. No wonder we use the term "cuckoo" to denote a bit of craziness in one's erratic actions.

Raising orphaned animals

Sometimes a member of one species will raise an orphaned newborn of another species or of its own. Often special techniques must be used to graft the two individuals together so the nursing dam does not smell an unwanted newborn. Sheep have a strong affinity for their own offspring and will always reject one from another ewe. However, if a lamb dies and a piece of its hide is tied to an orphaned lamb, the ewe whose lamb died will accept the orphan. Smell is a strong sense among animals. They recognize others more by smell than by sight. However, female dogs often accept species other than their own just by having the newborn brought to nurse. Dogs have been observed raising piglets, rabbits, kittens, coyotes, wolves, and many other species, including herbivores, in this manner.

Some scientists theorize that the domesticated dog evolved from wolves as a result of primitive women nursing orphaned wolf pups and taming them in the process. The history of domestication of animals is interesting. Domestication of the dog reportedly occurred 15,000 to 30,000 years ago, the goat 10,000 years ago, while most other animals were domesticated within the past 5,000 years.

While living in Maryland, I saw a giant woodpecker, (the pileated, *Hylatomus pileatus*), a spectacular bird with a red hood. This species is depicted in cartoons as Woody the Woodpecker. Its cartoon call is not at all like the sound made by the pileated woodpecker.

When I was 4 years old, visiting our friends the Schultz family on a Sunday afternoon, I entered their pig barn, climbed the supports that held the low-hung roof rafters, and discovered a mud-dauber swallow nest. The eggs in it were a bright blue. I brought one into the house, and Mr. Schultz said "Gordon, where did you get that bird egg?" I replied, "In yooor peeg hous."

I have been attracted to domesticated pigeons (*Columba livia domestica*, of which there are several breeds). Living in Davis in the mid-1970s, I maintained a small flock of barnyard-type homing pigeons, some of which were blue-gray with two black wing stripes; others were all white; and some were all black with fluorescent feathers in the neck area. Since 1993, when we moved to Dixon, the flock has grown to 30 or 40 birds that I use to train hunting bird dogs. Pigeons were domesticated in Egypt 5,000 years ago for use as message carriers. They are found in cities and towns in Europe, Asia, and the Americas. Pigeons seem to follow people, like types of rodents. I have seen them perched on the shoulders of people sitting in parks, often near large fountains that sound like natural waterfalls. Gregarious, they stay together in flocks that number into the hundreds.

My pigeons home (return) to their pen through a coned entrance. They must be shown once and helped through the entrance; thereafter they never forget how to enter. If they are not trained to enter, a few figure out how to get in. Such birds will hang around the pen area for a few days and then disappear, or take up roosting in a barn nearby. Those that disappear may join other flocks or may be caught by hawks or owls.

Most animals, after being taught a task, never forget. In contrast, much of human learning comes through repetition. Animals may need reinforcement in being taught various performance tasks. If an animal wants to escape captivity, it needs only once to figure out how to find a hole in an enclosed area or how to get over or under a barrier. A bad or painful experience is always remembered and often becomes a chronic fault in animal working endeavors. In U.S. field-trialing dogs under judgment, a dog wagging its tail on point is heavily faulted. In many such cases, the dog during training was painfully corrected while pointing a bird and never forgot that experience. As a result it will always experience anxiety and wag its tail on point.

Other animals

The first time I observed American bison (*Bison bison*), also known as the American buffalo, was on a trip to North Dakota with my grandparents in 1942 to visit Aunt Florence, who worked as a nurse in Minot. She took us out to dinner, and I had the opportunity to order a buffalo steak. It was lean, fairly dry, and delicious.

Bison belong to the *Bovidae* family, which includes true antelope, gazelles, wild and domestic cattle, sheep, goats, and water buffalo. The American bison numbered in the millions and ranged at one time over a large area of North America. Due to hunting, they were nearly exterminated in the late 19th century. Since then, they have increased in number, and several herds are protected in national parks and preserves. Few herds are genetically pure bison. There are only three free-roaming and genetically pure American bison herds on public lands in the United States. Most others have genetic relationships with domesticated cattle, through the female line. Commercially bred hybrids have been raised to provide a restaurant specialty meat referred to as beefalo. Our grandson Joshua, who works as a chef, orders beefalo that is one-third buffalo and two-thirds Angus beef to serve various meat dishes.

Wild North American felines

North American mountain lions and bobcats are secretive, allowing few opportunities to observe them in the wild. These *Felidae* are sleek and fast. Interestingly, their movements and actions are similar to those of domesticated cats. The mountain lion (puma) rarely attacks human beings. The only real threat comes when a den with kittens is approached. For her offspring's protection, a queen will attack a human, especially if the human sees the lion and runs away.

Bobcats are born with a shortened or hardly observable tail. Its domestic counterpart, the Manx cat, has a similar bobbed tail. Bobcats are inquisitive, and when seen in heavy cover will stare and look at a human if the human does not move. They are not dangerous to humans, however; after a few minutes, the cat will slowly turn and carefully walk away. The interesting genetic fact about the Manx cat is that the bobbed tail is a dominant gene. A homozygous pairing (with a gene for short tail from each parent) is lethal, and the developing embryos die in utero. Carolyn and I have a pet Manx that looks similar to a wild bobcat. Since it has a short tail, her name is "Bob." She is an affectionate and lovable cat.

Deer family

Deer, elk, and moose belong to the deer family, *Cervidae*. Deer are quiet and investigative. They scare easily and yet have enormous curiosity, a trait that allows them to come fairly close to humans who are standing, sitting, or otherwise being still. Quick movements will cause them to flee.

Bottle-raised deer fawns become tame and reside around where they were kept and raised as an infant. Strains of deer encountered in the United States include the white-tail deer found east of the Mississippi River and the mule deer inhabiting territory from the Rocky Mountains westward. The smaller black-tail deer, about half the size of mule deer and white-tails, resides along the West Coast, while the Pacific deer ranges mostly in California's coastal San Luis Obispo County. I once shot a Pacific deer. Mature Pacific deer never develop antlers beyond a fork, whereas other deer add tines or spikes to their antlers as they age.

Elk are members of the deer family and are similar in behavior. In rut (mating season), an elk bull can be called by a hunter using a device imitating a competing bull's call. Bulls will come as close as 10 yards from the person who has called, especially if the person is camouflaged and quiet. Elk are gregarious and are seen in large herds with several cows, some bulls, and calves. They look a lot like the European red deer (Hirsch) but are different species. North American elk are not found on other continents.

North American moose

The largest members of the deer family have huge antlers. They like marshy areas and are strong swimmers. In 1962, while visiting my sister, Blythe, and her family at Wonder Lake near Mount McKinley (now Denali) National Park in Alaska, I saw a moose swim with ease across Wonder Lake, a distance of five miles. Moose will forage the bottom of streams, lakes, and swamps for grass and plant life not easily found on the surface. While walking along a creek during an elk hunt in Idaho, I came across a very large bull moose that followed me from the other side of the stream for at least 30 minutes. He acted just like a domesticated cattle bull. Seeing this huge animal as close as 15 yards for many minutes created a vivid memory. Moose occur in northern Scandinavia, as well as in North America, and there are called elk. Despite the difference in names, they are the same species.

Antilocapridae

Pronghorn antelope are not *Cervidae* or deer family. Their horns are permanent, in contrast to deer, which annually shed their antlers. Pronghorns are members of the family *Antilocapridae.* Although eight species existed prehistorically in North America, only one remains in the United States. Pronghorns' main safety net is speed, and individuals can be easily incited into rapid acceleration topping 55 miles per hour. Pronghorns, too, have a sense of curiosity. If one lies prostrate on the ground and waits, an animal will come extremely close out of curiosity.

An overview of animal sociology

Animal trainers take advantage of the ability of animals to remember experiences. Training should be done in a way that is not foreign to the animal's ability to remember, and with reward in mind. Delmar Smith, known bird-dog trainer and author, gets it right when he says, "When training a dog, you have to think like a dog and read the dog's body language."

A veterinarian must understand the nature of the species and the individual in order to communicate. My father was such a gifted expert in training horses that he would purchase a horse that had never been touched by human hands, right off the prairie. Within a short time he would have a halter on the horse, have it follow him, and lead it behind a Model T Ford a few miles to its new home. The horse soon would become a member of a team that worked in a harness pulling farm implements.

Animals will exhibit fear if a veterinarian is attempting to hold or restrain it. They have the ability to read the human mind. The next strongest sense is that of touch. Petting or stroking and saying, in a quiet, reassuring voice, "What a good girl (or boy, cat, dog, or horse)" has a calming effect. The first experience most newborn or hatched animals have is touch from the dam or hen. Infants are cuddled, pushed around with the nose, and continually licked to stimulate urination and defecation or to be groomed. Chicks are sat upon to be kept warm. Touch is an amazing sense in animals as well as humans, so it should come as no surprise that animals like to be touched. Yet many veterinarians immediately start to examine the patient by sticking a thermometer up its anus, or taking out a stethoscope to listen to the heart and lungs. They should take an initial few seconds to greet the patient or gently touch it while getting acquainted. The first step in any examination of an animal, whether individual or part of a herd, is to become acquainted. The next steps then become easy. A caring veterinarian must be able to read the animal to be examined, and must show a feeling of compassion for animals at all times. Often during my career while examining animals, an owner of a cat or dog would tell me, "You are the first person other than one in our family who could touch Suzie."

Shangri-La, our vacation home

Our vacation home in Mendocino County always has been a special, God-given spot to relax and recharge in nature. The home is off Highway 1 on a steep hillside about a third of a mile from the gorgeous Mendocino coast and a mile north of Anchor Bay. In this region huge virgin redwood trees, some of them 1,000 or more years old, reach 200 feet and higher up to the heavens. Such trees on our property grow on the sides of a coastal canyon with a year-round creek. From our living-room window, they frame a view of the Pacific Ocean. In addition to natural beauty, the locale has an ideal climate: mildly warm in summer and cool but not cold in the winter months.

Our rustic vacation home was built in 1946 on the edge of the canyon. It is surrounded by numerous varieties of grasses and bushes, most of which become dormant during the dry summer months. Their foliage turns golden and emits a mixture of aromas that blend pleasantly with salty sea air. Sea lions can be heard barking at a nearby small island, Fish Rock, about 50 yards offshore.

Carolyn, our three children, and I fell in love with this very special place in 1970. It reminded us of the idyllic settings depicted in James Hilton's 1933 novel *Lost Horizon.* Is there any wonder why we call it Shangri-La?

A few years after we purchased our property, the water well's steel pipe system collapsed from rust, requiring a new well to be drilled. Recalling my experience in 1942 at Lake of the Woods, Minnesota, when I was introduced to water-witching techniques, I sought a person with such skills to locate a site for a new well at Shangri-La. Mrs. Warner, who lived only three miles away, used the same willow forked-stick technique I had observed as a young teenager. Sure enough, at the spot where the branch in Mrs. Warner's hands bent and twitched, water was found 120 feet below the surface. Ever since, even during the driest of years, the well has always been sufficient for our needs. The water is slightly red in color and has a faint, rusty aroma due to heavy iron content, but it tastes good and adds a good flavor to culinary endeavors.

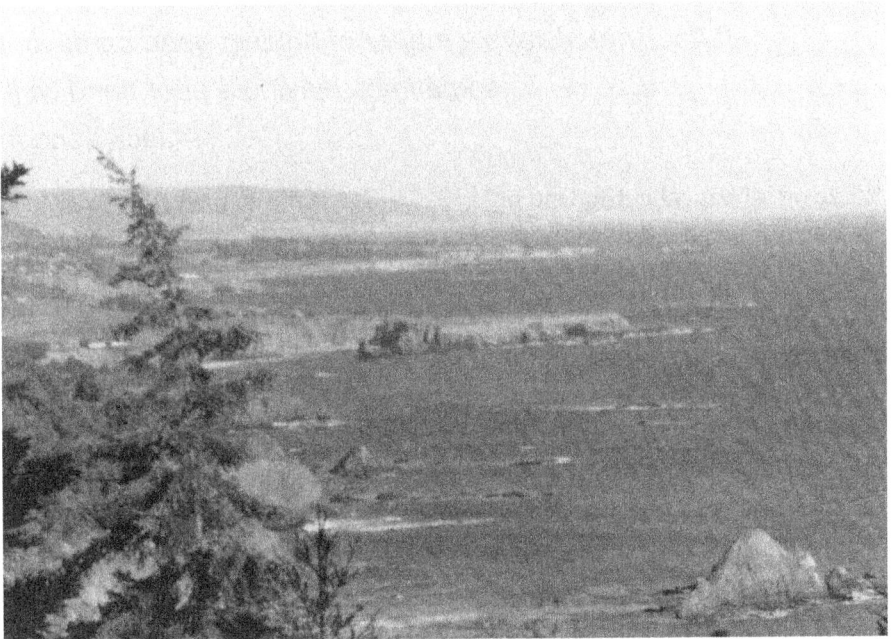

The view from our vacation home in Mendocino County.

CHAPTER 22

The Mystery of Multiple Sclerosis

"Life is not always a matter of holding good cards, but sometimes playing a poor hand well.
– Jack London

While on sabbatical in England in 1972–73, Carolyn experienced unexplained double vision and felt ill for weeks. By the time we prepared for our departure to Germany in 1979, she was definitively diagnosed with multiple sclerosis. She had flare-ups and improvements over the course of many years, but fortunately, she did not have a flare-up while we were in Germany.

Carolyn began seeing a neurologist in 1980. Sometime in the early 1990s, she first saw Mark Agius, M.D., at the UC Davis Medical Center in Sacramento. She remained under his care as her disease gradually worsened until a new drug, Copaxone, was prescribed. This drug held back life-threatening exacerbations, and since 1990 she has experienced a slowly progressive malady with no extreme flare-ups.

The first recorded person to suffer from MS was a woman named Halldora living in Iceland in the year 1200. She had one of the classical first signs of MS – sudden loss of eyesight that returned sometime later. Along with vision problems, she experienced weakness in her legs, clumsiness in movements of her hands, body numbness, and dizziness. Another woman, Lidwina, a nun who lived from 1380 to 1417 in Holland, developed the same traditional symptoms of MS but experienced improved health from the age of 16 until she died at 53. Lidwina had a form of MS that resulted in chronicity with relapses. In 1890 Pope Leo III declared her Saint Lidwina of Schiedam, the patron saint not of MS, but rather of ice skaters.

Multiple sclerosis had not yet been established as a disease. The "multiple" in the name refers to the scarring and changes of the nervous system it

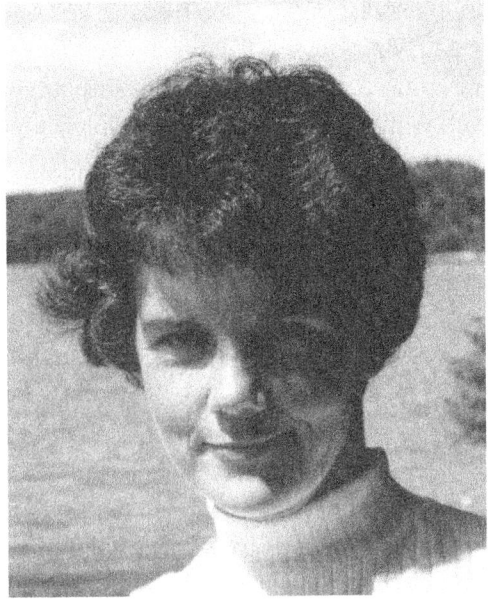

Carolyn at age 33 in Gull Lake, Minnesota, in 1964, before signs of MS became obvious.

induces in multiple parts of the body, from the brain to the extremities. Multiple sclerosis, which can progress slowly, is caused by an autoimmune reaction that triggers the body to destroy the neurolemma (covering of nerve sheaths), resulting in hindrance of nerve impulses from the brain to striated muscle and return of signals to the brain, preventing the nerve impulse from functioning as desired. The cause has not been identified. It occurs much more frequently in women than in men, and in people who live in countries and climates distant from the equator.

Even though no evidence of direct genetic inheritance has been found, MS does occur within familial relationships, which is true in Carolyn's family. Carolyn's second cousin Jacqueline du Pré, a famous cellist, and a first cousin, June Poole, had the disease, and all have family origins on the Island of Jersey in the English Channel. MS occurs with high frequency in the Channel Islands.

A scientist with expertise in slow-acting viruses could speculate that MS also is caused by a slow-acting virus, or perhaps a slow-acting protein like the prion protein that causes human and animal spongiform *encephalopathy* seen in Creutzfeldt-Jakob disease, kuru and mad cow disease. My experience of studying bovine leukemia virus and the inability of scientists to isolate the virus despite its constant presence tell me that might be happening as well with the elusive cause of MS. The putative agent always is present, but researchers have not been able to identify the precise cause of the disease. MS stimulates lymphocytes to damage nerve tissue that is needed for various bodily functions. Researchers must undertake good, sound, innovative MS causal research using novel approaches focused on finding the evasive source that triggers the disease.

Carolyn's first signs of a neurologic disorders were little different from the women in the Middle Ages in Iceland and Holland. Before the birth of our daughter, Ann, Carolyn experienced tingly and restless legs and feet when she was 25 years old. After Ann's birth, these symptoms continued, and Carolyn developed signs of pressure on the side of her body. While walking along she would suddenly fall. This occurred infrequently over a period of several years, with lapses in between that convinced me she simply was clumsy. When Ann was 17, before she graduated from high school, she traveled with Carolyn to visit several universities. On a trip to Cal Poly State University in San Luis Obispo and the University of California, Santa Barbara, Carolyn suddenly found herself unable to swallow. That condition lasted for one day.

Carolyn saw an internist at the Woodland Memorial Clinic for a number of years in the 1960s. Despite several visits during which she described the signs similar to those of the women who lived in the Middle Ages, the internist could find nothing wrong. He insinuated that these strange tingles and feelings of pressure existed only in Carolyn's imagination – or that she was neurotic. His opinion discouraged Carolyn from continuing to see him.

While I was on sabbatical at the Royal Marsden Hospital in England, Carolyn developed double vision and loss of balance with vertigo. This led to diagnosis as a middle-ear infection or Ménière's disease. She was treated for motion sickness and fatigue. This episode lasted for several weeks. When she returned to the United States, she again consulted internists – who remained unable to identify a specific cause.

In the spring of 1979, Carolyn was auditing a German language class at UC Davis in preparation for a year of living in Germany. I was at a World Health Organization meeting in Geneva and called home to check on how things were going. Carolyn had experienced double vision again. Covering one eye with her free hand in order to see a straight line on the road, she drove alone 10 miles to the Woodland clinic to see our ophthalmologist. He diagnosed optic nerve neuritis and inflammation of the retina, and referred her immediately to a neurologist, who did a spinal tap. On the basis of the ophthalmological finding and increased white blood-cell count in the spinal fluid, and history, the neurologist diagnosed MS as the cause of her symptoms. Before the diagnosis was made, Marilyn Herrmann, a good friend and a member of Davis Lutheran Church, was having similar signs. She told Carolyn that her doctors thought she had MS. Carolyn replied, "I have the same symptoms, and I doubt that you have MS because I do not have it." Wow!

The joy of the MS diagnosis

Carolyn related her diagnosis to me on the phone while I was in Geneva. She was overjoyed and elated that finally, after more than 25 years, a diagnosis had been made. It was a relief for her to know that she had a physical medical problem and not an emotional one. After all those frustrating years of not knowing the cause of her discomfort and unusual clinical changes, she finally had a conclusive answer.

Preventive therapy, and the slow progress of MS

Upon return from Geneva, I instituted passive immunotherapy by collecting 20 cc's of unclotted blood from Carolyn and injecting it intradermally into a pregnant cow. I had evidence in treating cancer patients with immunotherapy that best results were obtained by intradermal injection of vaccines. It is now known that this route of injection stimulates dendritic cells, initiating immune recognition of unwanted antigens. I repeated the procedure 10 days later.

When the cow gave birth, I collected colostrum (an initial mammary gland secretion) and froze it in 20 cc aliquots (samples). Carolyn took the medication daily for several weeks before we went to Germany in 1979. While there, she had no signs of MS and would daily run in the forest next to our apartment. Upon our return to Davis, she continued to walk every day with a friend, Lynn Campbell, but stopped bicycling due to balance problems. Whether the passive immunotherapy was beneficial was not documented. Saint Lidwina had a prolonged, chronic, relapsing form of MS similar to what Carolyn has experienced. Lidwina could have been exposed to a form of passive immunotherapy accidentally rather than planned as in Carolyn's situation.

Carolyn started using a wheelchair for long distances in place of a cane or walker. She experienced her first huge loss of independence following a minor car accident that made her realize that driving was dangerous. That resulted in an unbelievably huge change in lifestyle, and as MS has slowly progressed over time she has endured one loss of independence after another. Personal happiness is always associated with freedom to do as one wants to do. Throughout the past 40 years, Carolyn has been an angel and has never complained once about her state of health or wondered aloud about why she is so afflicted.

She used a cane and then a walker around the house and for shopping. In 2009 while descending steps, she fell onto cement flooring with a blow to the occipital (lower back) region of her head. From that time on, she has never taken stairs up or down without assistance from another person. During the spring of 2009 she had many falls. In May of that year she became fully reliant on a wheelchair, and transfers from her wheelchair to a reclining chair, bed, and toilet.

In February 2010, Carolyn began physical therapy by walking with a parachute-type harness similar to the one I wore in the 82nd Airborne in 1946–1948. In addition, she used a treadmill for exercises under the guidance of physical therapist Bryan Padilla. This exercise enabled her to resume walking again with the aid of a walker and a belt. Carolyn is elated every time she takes a short assisted walk.

No corticosteroid therapy

Progression from the first signs of the disease in the 1960s was slow, which I attribute, in part, to refusal of corticosteroid therapy during flare-ups. Injections of Copaxone have proved to be an extremely beneficial therapy. This drug, made up of three amino acid polymers and given daily for 10 years, has subdued exacerbations to a minimum. New research efforts are focusing on improved immunotherapy.

Carolyn may have had a low-grade experience with MS from the time we were married, because she was clumsy in running, throwing a softball, and in other activities. Nevertheless, in 50 years I have had ample opportunity to adjust to living with a person with MS. Little emotion has transpired between us on this matter.

Whenever I or a pastor or someone else said healing prayers or a special blessing for her, she said that she felt better and had a stronger desire to overcome MS handicaps. She prays daily to the Lord Jesus Christ, asking for strength. It is obvious that persons with a strong faith and strong support from family members and friends do well, yet in the National Multiple Sclerosis Society little or nothing is publicly said about the power of Christian prayer. The society endorses yoga and other Eastern exercise and meditation practices while generally overlooking one of the most powerful resources, Christianity and the power of prayer.

It has been difficult to accept the insidiousness of the slowly developing disease that has taken its toll, both physically and mentally, on an exceptionally talented individual. Her loss of short-term memory and her increasing need for assistance in daily tasks has been distressing. With aging, the fading of youth is expected. What is not expected is cognitive loss of mind and physical handicapping of the body as seen in MS. The power of God through daily prayer helps overcome the intensifying effects of neurological damage experienced with the disease.

Persons living without chronic maladies such as MS should be eternally grateful for what they have. Good health brings a brightly shining light in one's life. It takes enormous courage to daily confront loss of memory and physical abilities, and to cheerfully and positively survive with the malady for more than half a century.

CHAPTER 23

Retirement, 1993

"It ain't over 'til it's over."
– Yogi Berra

Our move from Davis to the countryside three miles away, north of the town of Dixon, was a transition that started in November 1991 and concluded a year later. It was difficult for Carolyn to leave friends in Davis, especially our neighbor Lynn Campbell. Carolyn and Lynn took morning walks together and were close companions.

While Carolyn was still driving she went to a health care facility on East 8th Street to visit her mother, Doreen MacMillan, who lived there for seven years. She and her husband, Ewell, could no longer care for themselves. Carolyn's visits became less frequent after she stopped driving. Paying for home health care had drained their life savings. Ewell moved in with his daughter, Martha, in San Leandro. He died in 2003 at age 91, and Doreen died two years later at the same age.

For thirty-seven and a half years the demands of remaining current in my profession required me to carry a briefcase and work whenever a free moment occurred, even at night and weekends, and to travel frequently by plane or train. My retirement from the University of California, Davis, began on January 1, 2003. During the five years that followed, I had difficulty weaning myself from the longtime pattern of remaining current in professional interests. The briefcase still remained with me, despite reduced urgency to finish a document. Recording thoughts by having new information available in a briefcase at most times helped me stay current. New textbooks or nonfiction books were in the briefcase for a quick read.

Having reading or writing material readily available during nearly four decades of employment helped me in manuscript preparation. Professional commitments could not be met in an eight-hour workday. I read hundreds and hundreds of books, my favorites among which were historical novels. Reading about a person, animal, geographic location, political thinking, or religious philosophies brought pleasureful gain in knowledge. A keen interest of mine has been leadership from ancient to modern times, and reading on that subject has given me insights into most influential leaders and how they helped shape historical events.

The greatest leader in all history is Jesus Christ, who came into the world amid humble surroundings as his mother, Mary, birthed him in a stable in the crowded city of Bethlehem. He in three short years of ministry developed a following that led to selection of 12 disciples. After his death, many new disciples and apostles helped spread his leadership in ministry to most of the known world. This all occurred within less than a hundred years. Thousands of leaders have followed his example, as have billions of followers who were baptized or converted to Christianity.

Reverence for Christ's leadership comes from a new and continued moral ethic that meant it mattered how one lives life, understanding God who is in control. It also matters that one who follows Christ's ministry understands and accepts that his teaching is the Word of God. His word preserved in the Holy Bible helped shape my leadership and that of thousands of other important research leaders, from antiquity to the present. Medical geneticist Francis S. Collins, principal investigator of the human genome project, wrote an exemplary 2007 book, *The Language of God: A Scientist Presents Evidence for Belief.*

Retirement ended the need to keep a rigid schedule and start the day's activities at a specified time. We made plans well before retirement to improve the 20 acres of land that we purchased near Dixon. The property included three homes, a 100-year-old redwood barn, a metal-roofed, 160-foot-long equipment building, and a three-stall horse barn. We dug a trench to extend underground electrical wiring from the old barn to the equipment building. We converted a portion of the equipment and machinery shed into an indoor-outdoor dog kennel with a grooming room and bathroom. The septic system was already established and was connected from the dog kennel area behind the old redwood barn.

The barn had a dilapidated aluminum roof, which we replaced with corrugated metal roofing. It had an unfinished barn loft apartment that was completed by Bob Anderson and John Lynn, who helped us with many projects to bring the property up to snuff. They became good friends, and Bob and his wife, Claudia, are in frequent contact. Bob, who is in his 80s, remains available for carpentry projects when needed. The property includes a large, manmade lake that was full of cattail tules and discarded slabs of cement. The previous owner was a building contractor and for some reason used the pond as a dump. It was a huge eyesore, at least to me.

During the first summer, Francisco Garcia, a capable young immigrant from Mexico, worked to help beautify the lake. He constructed a picturesque border of cement blocks that had been mechanically split from the numerous cement slabs in the lake. Francisco placed the cement blocks end on end next to 8-by-16-inch, chemically treated fir planks around three sides of the lake.

We used sixteen acres to grow and harvest grass hay for two horses and a riding mule. The property has been maintained with the help of several people, notably Sr. Bonifacio Nuñez, who since the mid-1990s has been the lead person assisting in day-to-day maintenance. The Nuñez family helped in many ways. Bonifacio's son Carlos, his wife, Elvia, and daughters Minerva and Henalise, aided Carolyn in housework. The ladies prepared delicious Mexican cuisine highlighted by a special chile relleno recipe. The work projects were always numerous, and need for reroofing, siding repair, and painting meant mainte-nance on an ongoing basis. The lake held water year-round for the first few years, then drought conditions led to total evaporation and loss of largemouth bass and feeder fish. Neighborhood kids used to fish for bass and release them.

Wildlife

Three acres that we set aside for wildlife habitat abound in bird and plant life. We dedicated it to planting native trees, shrubs, and grasses, preserving land for special flora and fauna found in the Sacramento Valley. I was proudly

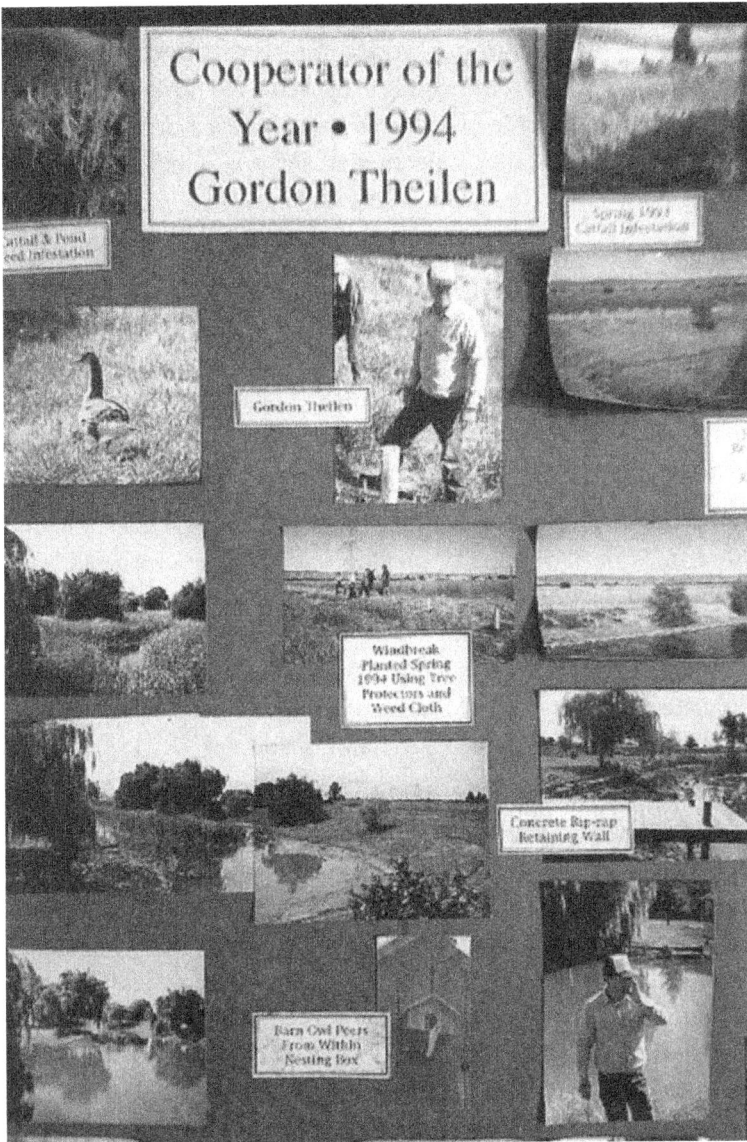

Cooperator of the Year poster depicting accomplishments in planting trees, shrubs, and grasses.

awarded the Cooperator of the Year Award in 1994 from Solano County and the USDA in recognition of our work to preserve natural habitat land. This was a new venture in the life of the Boy With the Wounded Thumb, and a fun project. Various native plants provided a source of seeds that attracted an abundance of animal life. Wild creatures can live there as they did before widespread cultivation changed the landscape.

Our retirement home has been a residence of love and seclusion among beautiful trees, including coastal redwoods and Australian pine (*Casuarina equisetifolia*), commonly called ironwood. The name is a combination of the Latin root words *equi* meaning "horse with bristles" and *folia* meaning "leaf." The foliage mimics a horsetail and gets its name from that description. A Roman who was referred to as Piney the Elder used the word "equisetum" in his writings in 40 A.D. to denote a horse's tail; thus *equisetum folia* means "horsetail-like leaf."

Other trees on the property include various species of oak, elders, and beautiful weeping willow trees with gorgeous branches sweeping to lake level. Scrubs of many kinds are sprinkled among more than 100 trees – wonderful fig, persimmon, orange, lime, tangerine, grapefruit, kumquat, tangelo, and pomegranates, which evoke the feeling of being in forest rather than surrounded by thousands of acres of farmed agricultural land.

Birds abound as part of the wildlife habitat. Barn owls (*Tyto alba*) reside on the property and hoot at night, particularly during a full moon. Because they are nocturnal and stay secluded in the daytime, we rarely see them. They have a nesting box near the point of the roof on the west side of the old barn and another nest on the rafters in the high-beamed hay barn. Black-hooded night heron (*Nycticorax nycticorax*) come every November and remain until February, when they migrate to southern Canada. A flock has established a rockery in the trees surrounding the lake. They know I will not molest them, and they rarely fly in my presence. However, when strangers approach, they fly a distance to stay safe. They roost in the daytime and forage at night. When darkness falls, they fly off one by one to feed in nearby swampland, and return at dawn to stay as secluded as possible, hiding in the branches of the weeping willow trees.

Common egrets (*Casmerodius albus*), seen along irrigation canals and wetlands in the surrounding areas, roost at night in our backyard redwood trees. Cattle egrets (*Bululcus ibis*), smaller white birds, do the same. When they come in at night to roost, there is a ruckus for several minutes until the birds' territory in the tree is established. Cattle egrets are seen in summer months among cattle grazing in nearby pastures. They stand on cattle that are lying down, catching flies in what is clearly a summertime symbiotic relationship between the two species.

Canada geese (*Banta Canadensis*) also nest around the lake, usually only one pair. They hatch on the average four goslings and enjoy the seclusion of the area. The family group does not return, but every other year what apparently is the same pair returns to nest. Mallard ducks (*Anas platyrhynchos*) nest near the lake each spring, and often two hens lay eggs. In contrast to the geese, the drake leaves the hen after mating, and she raises the youngsters by herself. The gander always stays with the goose. What is good for the gander is always good for the goose, but the drake doesn't do much good for the hen.

Ever since neighbors planted English walnut trees in 2013, wild turkeys (*Meleagrididae*) have increased to number around 50. Some hens nest along the secluded areas of the lake bank, and we have observed hatches of 10 or more. These birds nest in trees and forage on the back lawn. An interesting behavior not seen in other species relates to certain hens that act as lookouts and sentinels to protect the flock from impending danger. The hen of the hatch teaches the young to roost by flying into trees, with the young following her. The young can fly soon after hatching, but must sleep under the hen for warmth until plumage is sufficient to maintain body heat when roosting.

Ring-neck pheasants (*Phasianus colchicus*) have been present and increased in number with the new habitat. The influx of large numbers of turkeys create conflict over territory, resulting in fewer pheasants. California quail (*Lophortyx californicus*) have recently established a covey, and some nearby coveys come to our area for short periods of time. They bring memories of time when they numbered in the thousands on habitat that no longer exists, except our few acres.

Mourning doves (*Zenaidura macura*) abound in the habitat and always migrate south in the winter. Their cooing and mourning sound is heard morning and evening. These birds accentuate peace and tranquility in the surrounding area and give an inner appreciation of the wonders that God has given mankind. Birds help provide awareness of the gift given to live at such a wonderful place, a bit of heaven on Earth.

Other species of birds are present, and jackrabbits abound in the nearby fields. Hawks of various species are seen, and crows are abundant. Nearby resident pairs of crows act a bit tame, almost pet-like. Scrub blue jays, mockingbirds, and yellow-beaked magpies are numerous. Little songbirds migrate through spring and fall. A few hummingbirds present each summer bring to full light the wonder of how DNA was put together to enable living creatures to function in awesome ways. We have a small population of bats seen at dusk that reside in the old barn and shed, and migrate south in cooler months.

Home and garden

Our retirement home is spacious, with two bedrooms, one of which has a large walk-in closet and attached bath. Carolyn has full use of a remodeled bath with a wheelchair entry and accessible shower area. A study area opens onto the master bedroom at one end and dining area at the other. The living area is a large room with a wood-burning stove used to partially heat the house in winter. A nice, compact kitchen opens to the living room on one side and the laundry-utility area on the other. The entrance to the garage is through the laundry room.

Vegetable gardening is an every-summer activity. The garden provides fresh vegetables and several varieties of squash that are stored and used for winter month eating. I enjoy propagating herbs. Several are perennial, while a few, such as sweet basil, are annuals. We use these herbs profusely in cooking. Cucumber salad, a summer favorite of ours, is made from freshly sliced garden cucumbers, minced or sliced sweet red onions, garden-derived tomatoes, red wine vinegar, abundant freshly picked sweet basil, fresh pepper, and a pinch of salt. This salad was always served in the summertime at my great-aunt Gertie Theilen's home that I fondly remember from the early 1930s. Grandma Schaller also made cucumber salad each summer. Every time such salad is served, I flash back to my boyhood days in the 1930s.

Health conditions

Each year, in late winter and early spring, allergic reactions from tree and grass pollens bring on severe sneezing and difficulty in breathing. I experience first signs in late January and February from acacia tree blossom pollen. Wild grasses, other trees, and scrubs begin pollinating a month later, inducing frequent allergy attacks. Antihistamine medication and nasal mask protection help diminish my symptoms; adrenaline is always available to ward off anaphylaxis. In recent years, hundreds of acres of agricultural land adjoining the property have been planted in English walnut and almond trees, both of which increase allergy problems.

My affliction with advanced chronic osteoarthritis and low-grade pain in the lower back cause me discomfort 24 hours a day, seven days a week. My first morning activity is exercise. I lie on the floor stretching and pulling muscles and tendons to straighten bony structures. Exercise on stationary bicycle, which I pedal for 10 to 15 minutes, is helpful. Walking outside with a cane gives needed exercise while I care for a horse, "Chance," three dogs, chickens, and homing pigeons in the aviary. I use pigeons for dog training. The summer walks also include taking care of the vegetable garden, which bring my total outside walking to a half-mile or more each day.

In 2007, I underwent surgery to replace a longtime painful left knee joint, with quick recovery and relief. The following year, difficulty I experienced in breathing during exercise led to diagnosis of a major heart artery blockage, the anterior descending aortic arterial blood vessel. Implantation of a stent relieved the blockage, and rectified all related health problems.

A drug-related episode resulted in acute hemorrhage from inflammatory colitis and near death resulting from loss of more than 50 percent of my blood volume. I was immediately hospitalized and within 30 minutes, due to acute loss of blood, cardiac arrest occurred with severe chest pains and sudden unconsciousness. I awakened several hours later in intensive care with blood dripping into my arm. I immediately responded well to the blood transfusion. I was taken off all medications when it became obvious that one or more of them may have triggered the colon hemorrhage. This near-death episode occurred on April 1, 2009 – not a trick, but a real event. On March 28 I had undergone a colonoscopy during which two polyps were removed and diverticulitis was found. Two days later I had a tooth implant. The dental surgeon initiated medication with 500 mg of the antibiotic amoxicillin for five days. I was off Plavix, an anti-clotting drug, for four days before the colonoscopy, and began taking it again two days before the dental procedure.

On the fourth day of my amoxicillin regimen, I began having severe bloody diarrhea at 6 a.m. I immediately contacted my gastroenterologist, who told me

209

to see my general practitioner. I wound up seeing a substitute physician but not until late in the afternoon, after passing large amounts of blood numerous times during the day. At 5 p.m., I was instructed to collect a fecal sample for culture and come back the next day for a lab workup. I stressed that I needed a CBC (complete blood count) now. I should have gone across the street to the Emergency Department at Sutter Davis Hospital.

Ann had come to the UC Davis clinic to see me for another reason and said, "Dad, you look pale. Do you think you should drive"? I told her that I was OK, and then drove home in a weakened state, arriving there at 6 p.m. As soon as I entered our home, another bloody diarrhea episode led to a feeling of extreme weakness. I understood the gravity of so much blood loss and called a good friend, Sharon Jahn, who immediately took me to Woodland Hospital's Emergency Department. We arrived around 7:00 p.m. and the ER staff awaited my arrival. I had telephoned the on-duty gastroenterologist, who understood that immediate action was needed, and alerted the ER staff to be ready upon my arrival. I was placed on an IV drip within 15 minutes of our arrival. Soon after hospitalization I weakly walked to the toilet and passed a profuse amount of blood. I had severe chest pains and fainted in cardiac arrest.

Only after I had received four units of blood in the ICU did the hemorrhaging begin to stop. The original gastroenterologist who had done the colon exam a week earlier took me from the ICU for a diagnostic colonoscopy to determine the cause. The polyp removal area had no sign of ulceration and was not the cause of the hemorrhage, but nevertheless severe colon inflammation was found. I subsequently was diagnosed as allergic to amoxicillin, which had caused colitis and, in combination with Plavix, led to severe hemorrhage. This drug-related medical accident could have been prevented with proper use of an anticoagulant and knowledge of amoxicillin allergy.

Miracle in the Mojave Desert

In 2013, I again developed signs of tightness in the chest and shortness of breath while walking 100 yards. This led to the same concern had in 2007 before the arterial blockage was corrected with a stent. In November 2013, just before Thanksgiving, I was hospitalized for possible correction of stent problems. Tests revealed severe aortic valve insufficiency. Evaluation was considered for possible valve replacement by transcatheter at UC Davis Medical Center. I was placed on a waiting list and left in limbo. Christmas and New Year's Day came and went with no information about when the procedure would take place. The important benefits of using the transcatheter approach were quick delivery and avoidance of cutting and opening the chest cavity and heart.

The third week in January 2014, my good friend Christine Zink was participating at the San Diego Brittany Club Field Trial held on the California City grounds in the Mojave Desert. She was on her way to watch an event for energetic dogs that are keenly intent on finding game. On her way she passed the camp of fellow participant Bob West, and had a chat. Chris and I had known Bob for a several years and always talked about our common interest in dogs. In the course of the conversation Chris asked Bob "what is your line of work?" Bob replied "I work in the research department of Edwards Lifesciences in Irvine, California, and we make heart valves that are placed by transcatheter delivery." Christine told him, "Gordon needs aortic valve replacement and has been waiting more than two months for surgery." Bob said that his company had a clinical trial in progress at Stanford University Medical School using a newer version of the valve.

Bob asked, "Do you think Gordon would be interested?"

Chris replied, "Let's call him now."

When Chris called me, I immediately replied "YES."

Thus began my contact with Edwards Lifesciences. I was told to contact Dr. Craig Miller, who was in charge of the clinical trial. I called and made arrangements to have my medical history sent to Stanford. I was examined there in March and found to be suitable for assignment to the clinical trial. Hospitalization began on March 24 for insertion of a new valve into the femoral artery in my right groin, from which point it would be migrated for placement over the old valve in the heart. The surgery began at 7 a.m. March 25, and by 1 p.m. I was able to stand and with assistance get out of bed, sit in a chair and sip fluids. In four days the Boy With the Wounded Thumb was released from the hospital. On my one-month check-up, evaluation showed that the valve was perfectly functioning with no leakage.

The miracle in the Mojave that occurred by power of the Holy Spirit, prompting Chris to ask what Bob West did for a living, led to surgery at the skilled hands of Dr. Miller and his staff. This allowed me to continue to live a healthy life, complete this book, and present the keynote address, "One Medicine War on Cancer," at the World Veterinary Congress on May 25 in Iguassu, Brazil. The 429 registrants at the conference came from 27 countries on five continents. The specialty of veterinary cancer medicine established at the University of California, Davis, in the 1960s has evolved into a large international specialty, of which I'm exceptionally proud to be a part.

Establishment of a home church

Retirement gave me time to reflect on the gift of life and record what the Lord provided during 87 years. I was given the opportunity at age 84 to establish a home church along with Carolyn in 2012. It became a joyous endeavor that broadened my knowledge of Christianity and provided new ventures and Christian experiences.

We came to this decision after experiencing "progressive theology" and "Pharisaical theology" in association with national church body affiliations. This led to development of a Bible-oriented congregation. The Association of Free Lutheran Congregations provided an affiliation with an understanding that theology centers with truths found in the Holy Bible. The local congregation is the highest administrative authority. Importance of bible understanding and interpretation has been the norm with Israelite worshipers for 5,000 years and Christians for 2,000 years. We departed a congregation with continuous membership for 54 years and transferred to a conservative congregation for two years. In both congregations over that span of 56 years, we realized that parishioners are led by administrative authority beyond local congregation authority. We realized that church hierarchy is created by humans and their affiliated institutions rather than by God. This profound revelation led to a home church affiliated with the Association of Free Lutheran Congregations, which supports autonomy of each associated congregation.

God led us to establish a congregation that emulates the early Christian Church philosophy, the center of worship, the Word, and follows Christ's command to love God with all one's heart, mind and soul, and to love thy neighbor as thyself. This meant living Christianity daily around the clock, whatever one's everyday endeavor might be.

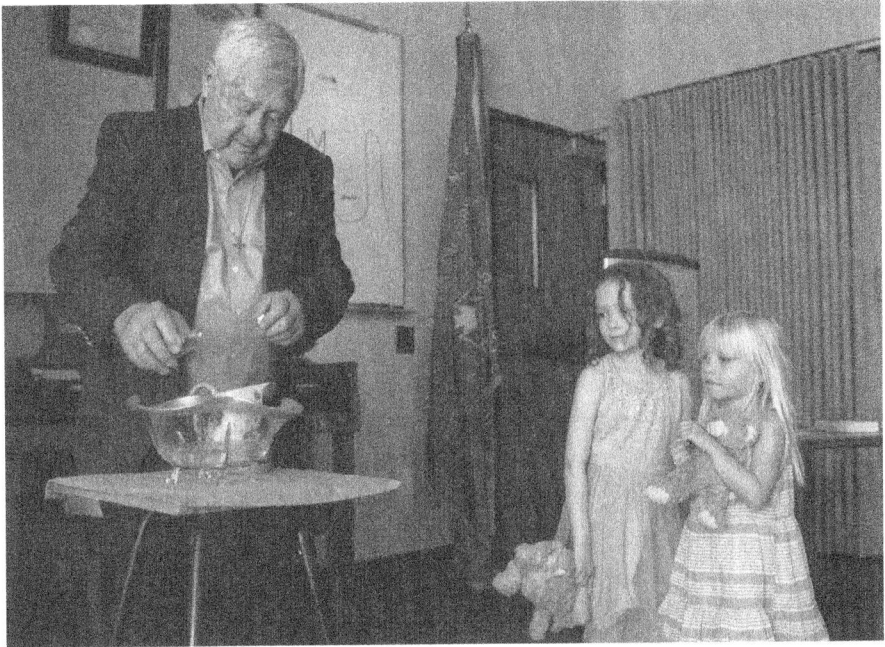

Jacquelyn and Zoe Theilen's baptism (Compliments of Matthew Theilen).

Our congregation developed a sound Christian constitution and doctrine established since the time of Christ's ministry and historically stressed by Augustine and reaffirmed at the time of the Evangelical Reformation in the early 1500s led by Martin Luther. In the Reformation, the early apostles emphasized that eternal salvation comes from belief in Christ as the only leader of the Church given in the Bible by His Word. We continue to stress Grace and Faith as provided in our doctrine.

As lay leader of the Home Church, the Boy With the Wounded Thumb has by the power of the Holy Spirit baptized eight people, bringing the miracle of becoming children of God. Holy Communion is conducted as done by early Christians in acceptance of Christ's real presence. Lessons for each church service follow a church-year calendar, with readings from the Old Testament, Psalms, Epistle and Gospel, lessons read and discussed by members of the congregation.

We are blessed to be among several hundred other Lutheran congregations affiliated worldwide with the Association of Free Lutheran Congregations (AFLC). This association provides participation in local and foreign mission outreach, youth and Bible College education, and help when needed to conduct Christian services in Dixon and surrounding communities. There is no church hierarchy, no synodical organization, and we at Dixon Trinity Free Lutheran are independent to conduct our services as we believe they should be. However, by our Constitution we are bound by an unchangeable doctrine as found in the Holy Bible and reaffirmed in the Evangelical Reformation of the 1500s established at Augsburg (known as Lutheran Confession) in 1530. That was,reaffirmed in the Book of Concord (Concordia, Latin for agreeing together) in 1580 in Dresden. Hundreds of theologians attended; Luther was at neither meeting. These documents soundly follow Christ's Word as found in the Holy Bible and form the basis for our independent congregation in Dixon free of church hierarchy.

CHAPTER 24

Purebred Hunting Dogs

"Dog is man's best friend."
– Frederick II, King of Prussia

I yearned as a 12-year-old for another dog after moving from Minnesota in 1939 to Richmond. I missed Rex and Tricksy. Soon after moving, I acquired a stray white female spitz-type cross. She was a good companion but with pups, and my parents insisted I could not keep her for monetary reasons.

The next dog I owned was in 1955 when we obtained a beagle from the beagle research colony at the UC Davis School of Veterinary Medicine. Dr. Anderson, the veterinary faculty director of the Laboratory for Energy-Related Health Research funded by the U.S. Atomic Energy Commission, provided our next dog. The study he directed determined long-term effects of radiation nucleotides exposure. He and his colleagues used adaptable laboratory-bred beagle dogs in their study. Breeding pairs provided puppies for lifetime studies. When the population of puppies exceeded research needs, extras were available for adoption.

We obtained a male puppy that we named "Lemmie." This pup came into our home shortly before we left to spend our year in Oregon. Lemmie was a typical beagle who freely explored the entire town of Tillamook. We did not have sufficient space for him and he was frequently tethered to the backyard clothesline near a doghouse. After setting up residence in Davis upon our return to California, Lemmie would wait to escape from the backyard and roam Davis. One day in 1970, he never came back, which led to acquisition of our first Brittany, a life-changing event in our relationships with dogs.

Hunting upland game birds

When I was a youngster in Minnesota, Dad found time each fall to hunt pheasants that were extremely plentiful because in the 1930s proper habitat was abundant. Pheasants originated in Manchuria. Dad would hunt with his nephews John and Edward Theilen from Minneapolis and with local friends, including Mr. Fred Schaeffer. After being involved in a job-related accident, Mr. Schaeffer became unable to hunt any longer. Dad acquired Mr. Schaeffer's 12-gauge Stevens pump shotgun, and 75 years later it is a showpiece in my home.

I was allowed to walk behind the hunting group who progressed in line going down harvested field corn rows between dried cornstalks. One or two hunters would wait at the end of the field as pheasants would mostly run ahead

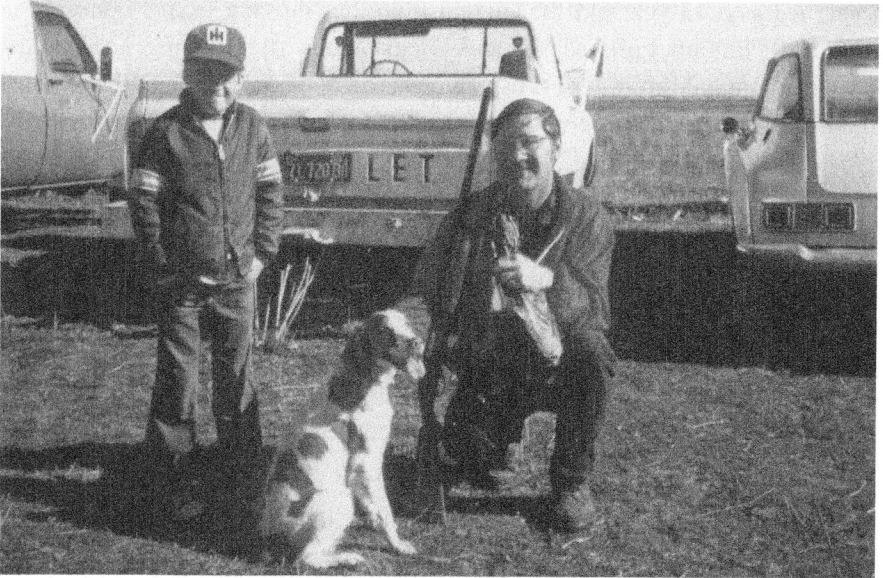

Darby's Dusty Lady in 1970 with the first pheasant shot over her, at Glide Tule Ranch in Yolo County, California. A young friend is with me in the picture.

216

out of shooting range until they became aware persons were ahead of them, and then they stopped. They were pushed to flight by those stalking through the field toward them.

As they took to flight, the hunters at the edge of the field fired at them. The birds that dropped had to be retrieved. Marking and finding downed birds was a task that took great effort, and some were not found. A dog to point and retrieve would have been helpful. We obviously needed a bird dog for hunting pheasants, but our family lacked the monetary resources to own another dog. The most needed dog was Rex, our German shepherd, who guarded our property and served as a pet.

My next opportunity to hunt pheasants came in November 1953, when I was a married student in veterinary school. My brother in-law, Mike, invited me to go pheasant hunting on Dixon farmland with a group of friends, including one fellow from Cayucos, California, who owned a black Labrador retriever. This dog opened my eyes for need of a retrieving dog to mark a downed game bird and bring it to hand. From that hunt, until purchasing my first hunting dog, a Brittany named "Dusty," I knew that a bird dog was a necessary hunting companion. She hunted pheasants with me in the Sacramento Valley for several pheasant seasons from November to early December.

Darby's Dusty Lady (AKC-SA921049)

I purchased Dusty from a Sacramento breeder who was recommended by one of my veterinary school classmates, Dr. Don Martinelli. The breeder was one of Don's clients. Don was a good source to obtain information about a Brittany because he owned two. Dusty's sire, Darby's Freckles D'Acajou II C.D, was a show obedience dog, and her dam, Suzanne's Dusty Lady (akc-SA530046), was a hunting dog.

Colleagues from the veterinary school and others enjoyed bird hunting. Our favorite hunting area was the Glide Tule Ranch 15 miles southeast of Davis. Dr. John Hughes, a colleague, was in charge of getting passes for permission to hunt on the Glide Tule Ranch for the season. The habitat for wild pheasants was as good as areas in South and North Dakota. The limit was two roosters per day. Our party usually consisting of 12 to 15 people went home with two pheasants each on opening day. A few other hunters also used hunting dogs, including the veterinary school's clinical pharmacist, Reed Enos, who had a trained German shorthaired pointer. Hunting with a bird dog enhanced my hunting experience and was a source of much joy.

Dusty, an orange-and-white colored dog, was a perfect year-round pet and a useful hunting dog for a few weeks out of the year. I had little time for hunting except during California pheasant hunting season. Dusty was a so-so pointer and marked the downed birds well, but failed to retrieve. This was not the perfect hunting dog I had wished for but it turned out she was the foundation bitch for our eventual establishment of Breton Kennels in Dixon to breed good hunting dogs.

Dusty loved being outside and never resisted going with us wherever we went anywhere on foot, by bicycle, or in the car. She adored being with kids, and her favorite outings were tent camping and backpack trips. She excelled in all types of camping activities, including playing catch with a ball and swimming in fast-moving mountain stream water. When it was time for us to go to sleep, Dusty would be found inside at the foot of the sleeping bag, asleep. She hated to be expelled to sleep on the outside, which obviously was not nearly as warm, and we always relented and let her sleep inside. She was a superb pet until she was killed in a car accident at 12 years of age. She was running across Fish Rock Road near our vacation home after I had called her to come. Wow, it was a sad day. Also coming to my call was her grandson, Luc, who luckily was not hit.

I also had taken Dusty when I went feral hog hunting. She was never far from my side, which was not acceptable for a pig hunting dog. Dusty would chase deer and always return in 15 to 20 minutes, the extent of her independence. As a hunting dog, she was of average motivation. While hunting hogs with Albert Gianoli, I saw the leader of his wild hog hunting dog pack. That Brittany impressed me enough to arrange mating with Dusty.

Gianoli's Pat (AKC-SB8526850)

Pat was an orange roan standard-sized Brittany with slightly bowed front legs. The term "roan" refers to areas of dominant color interspersed with hairs of another color. Pat was sired by Mister Chips XII (AKC SA388435) and out of Snow Bunny (AKC SA430162). Pat was versatile for bird, deer, and hog hunting. He excelled in retrieving game birds. When two wild pigeons were dropped and fell quite a distance from each other in a steep canyon,

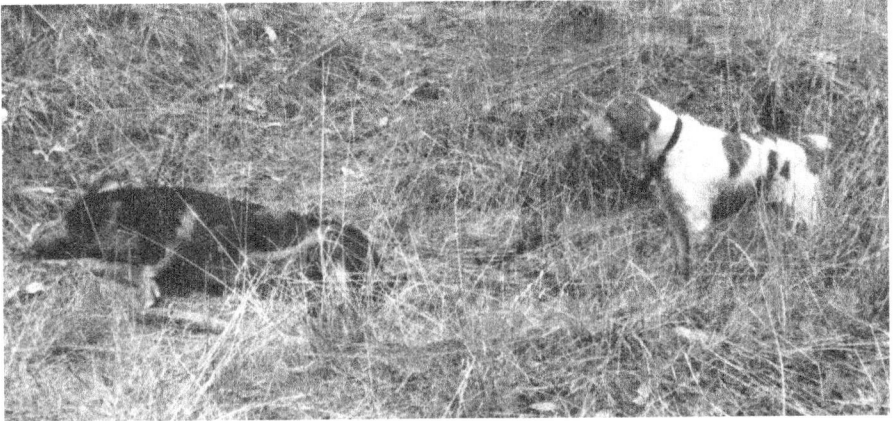

Luc Le Breton SH (AKC-SD600625) "Luc" pointing to a recently shot wild hog. This versatile Brittany was excellent as well in hunting upland game.

he retrieved two at one time, coming up a very steep canyon wall to bring the birds to hand. The selection of unique hunting traits has made our Breton Kennels dogs special and decidedly different from most American Brittanys in color selection and eagerness, coupled with boldness in hunting.

Pat knew that when Albert was walking with a shotgun, it was for hunting upland game and left hog scent alone. When with hunters riding horses with a scabbard attached to the saddle holding a rifle, and with other dogs as a pack, he ignored quail scent and instead followed hog scent like a hound. Pat with two or three other dogs would corner a pig and surround it when located. If it ran, they would nip at the heels and the hog would eventually seek protection by backing into a bush or tree and then would not move. Dogs would then bay like a hound. We would hear the dogs baying, perhaps miles away. After the hog was shot and killed, dogs would stay around as it was field dressed and attached to the saddle and the horse was mounted or walked back to camp. The dogs knew the hunt was over and would stay alongside the horses until reaching home, which might be as much as 10 miles from the site of the hog kill.

Pat's parents were registered Brittanys while the owner of Snow Bunny (who was mostly white with some orange) had not registered the litter at Pat's whelping. I helped Al Gianoli register Pat so we had a registered dog for Dusty's mating. She had a litter of eight wonderful, perfect pups, but due to Carolyn developing early signs of MS – notably fatigue – and not yet knowing what was wrong, we did not want to keep a pup. One female pup (Docca Severson) was

219

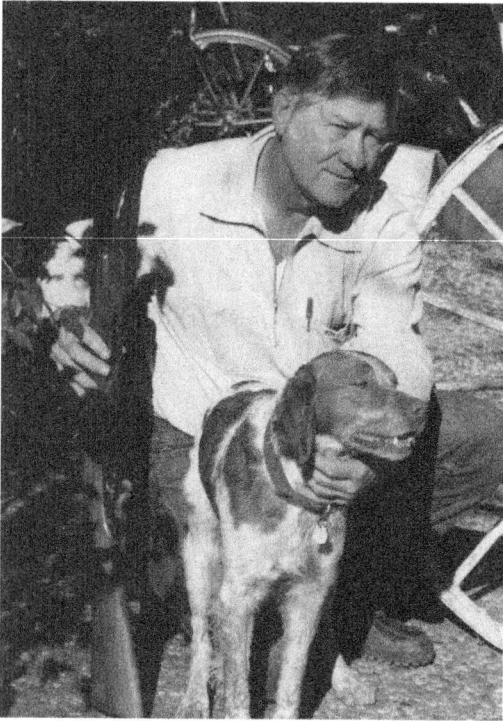

Luc with me after a pheasant hunt.

purchased by a friend, Charlie Marks, who worked at UC Davis Veterinary Medicine Central Services. The pup was an orange roan pointing and retrieving bird dog.

A few years later, Docca Severson was mated with Mister Bojangles XXXI. This orange-and-white male sire was a great-grandson of a famous dog, NAFC/DC/ AFC Tigre's Jocko, known as "Jocko." (For explanation of the title designations, see "Vocabulary of dog trials" in the Appendix.) From this litter, Carolyn agreed to keep a pup, which came to our home at 8 weeks of age. I had just arranged to travel as a guest of the French government to a special meeting in Paris on domestic animal cancer chemotherapy. I was required to travel by Air France because the French government paid for the trip. The travel agent's name was Luc and our little male orange roan pup was named Luc Le Breton.

He was introduced to hunting game at 6 months of age when he held point, and honored another dog on point (he looked like he was pointing the other dog). This inherited trait instinctively gave him manners to avoid disrupting another dog on point. As he aged he would hold point for up to 15 minutes or until the game moved and he was pointing an empty area. He was introduced to wild hog hunting at an early age, and by the time he was a mature dog became superb in scenting wild pigs.

His had great desire to hunt as pack leader for wild hogs in California coastal terrain. He would go with me and two or three other dogs, and stay near while hunting off horseback. When he detected the scent of wild hogs, he would run and follow the scent like a hound. He might be out of sound and sight for hours, later to be found baying a hog surrounded by other dogs. The hog would back into rocky or brushy areas to gain safety from the rear. These types of situations meant diligence in finding dogs as they would patiently await our arrival. They would stay surrounding the pig for hours, even overnight if not found during daylight hunting hours.

The miraculous amazing aspect of Luc's ability was that he was a versatile hunting dog as was his great grandfather, Gianoli's Pat. What a superb hunting dog, especially considering that he was self-taught. He was a pleasure to hunt upland game as he would figure out game conditions and how to approach game in different ways every time in the field. If pheasants, quail, or other upland game would run ahead, then stop, then go on for hundreds of yards, Luc developed a self-taught maneuver in which he did an end run around and went several hundred yards beyond running birds. He would stop them by cautiously walking back toward us. In that way he "pinned" the birds, which would flush as we approached within shooting range of about 25 yards. Luc would retrieve downed birds to hand, sometimes in multiple numbers. He always brought the bird to me, and perhaps others shot by fellow hunters. When I shot a double, Luc retrieved both.

Luc was a house pet when not hunting and would stay in certain sections of the house and never step onto the living room carpeting because he was trained to stay on uncarpeted areas, where he slept on bedding we provided for him.

These early experiences led to breeding Brittany Dogs that were bold and versatile in hunting all types of game. Dog breeding became a new fascination for me, one at the intersection of three loves of mine: veterinary care, hunting, and competitive field trials. I began breeding from the inquisitive perspective of a scientist, when I realized that I could make important contributions to the breed itself by selecting for improvements in genetic lineage. I embarked on that journey in 1970, detailed in the Appendix at the end of this book.

CHAPTER 25

Training, Genetic Selection, and Performance

"Tell me and I forget, teach me and I may remember,
involve me and I learn."
– Benjamin Franklin

Achievement of show and field championships is a high competition goal. People have for centuries claimed they had the best bull, ram, horse, or dog. During the Old Testament era people of Israel would sacrifice their prize oxen as an offering to God. This to them was the highest acknowledgement one could claim for a prized animal.

Dog selection that began in Victorian England for certain tasks led to different breeds of dogs. Brittanys were selected to serve as a family pet and a hunting dog. Selection for hunting traits and social behavior gave the Brittany special attention in the early 20th century. Training and environment are important for a Brittany to gain acclaim in competition. Development of a polished field dog happens after hours of training. Good, consistent exercise and a comfortable living environment help gain blue ribbons. The breed brought from France, L'Epagneul Breton, translates in English as Brittany.

L'Epagneul Breton

I decided that a pointing upland game dog of smaller size was for our home. The first hunting dog was chosen as a family project to become a pet and hunting dog. Some people erroneously refer to Brittanys as spaniels, but they are pointing dogs, not spaniels. Brittanys point game but look much like springer spaniels, especially Welsh springer spaniels, which do not point game. In response to the urging of the American Brittany Club, the American Kennel Club officially changed the name from Brittany spaniel to Brittany in 1970. The American Field Registry had always referred to the breed as Brittany.

At the Louvre in Paris, paintings from the 14th, 15th, and 16th centuries depict hunting dogs with short tails similar to the present-day Brittany, which often is born with a natural bob tail. I theorize early Celtic people brought such dogs with them from Indo-European areas centuries before the breed was recognized in 1906 at a certified Paris meeting. Callac, a small village in Bretagne, is historically the place of origin. A large bronze statue of a Brittany is found in the town square. A similar stature was erected in 2016 at the Bird Dog Field Trial Hall of Fame in Grand Junction, Tennessee, next to the Hall of Fame building.

Carolyn and I had the good fortune to visit Brittany breeders in 2006 and see French dogs up close. In October 1995, I wrote an article titled "From the Wolf to the Brittany," published in *The American Brittany* magazine. The article theorized that the Brittany was a unique breed of ancient origins. That study brought me to learn more about the Indo-European people, who were fond of animals. In 2012, my colleague Dr. Niels Pedersen, Hongwei Liu, Benjamin Sacks and I published a manuscript titled "The Effects of Dog Breed Development on Genetic Diversity and Relative Influences of Performances and Conformation Breeding" in the *Journal of Animal Breeding and Genetics*. In that study, we described a Brittany maternal Y-chromosome haplotype that had never been found before, even in more than 400 feral dogs from around the world, including Iran (ancient Persia).

Various reports and other breeds that my colleagues and I studied implied the genetic uniqueness of the Brittany. As hypothesized in an article I wrote on "Genetic defects committee reports from the wolf to the Brittany" for the *American Brittany Magazine* (Vol. 57, number 10, October 19, 1995), I declared the Brittany as genetically unique and different from all other hunting dogs. This was based on information other than genetic studies and certainly not from books written on the history of the breed.

Brittanys are the world's smallest pointing breed dogs, about the size of a standard cocker spaniel with longer legs. They have enormous energy and genetically are hunting dogs. The original breed had genetic traits that differed from all other pointing breed upland hunting dogs by possessing genes for pointing and retrieving whelped with a natural bobbed tail. The natural bob tail gene is dominant over a long tail. If a bob tail gene is inherited from both parents, the developing embryos die in utero before birth. This is a lethal gene combination that also exists in Manx cats.

Coat color of orange and white, liver and white, liver and white with orange highlighted (tricolor), or black and white are accepted as standard colors. Color patterns of subdued brownish buff (orange roan) or darkish liver (liver roan) or grayish black (black roan) exist over the standard hair colors.

Genetic selection

Brittany inheritance came from the wolf in a line of ancestors from the origin of the dog, according to scientific studies of what occurred from 15,000 to 25,000 years ago. The first domesticated dogs were working guard dogs to protect people, sheep, goats, and cattle from marauding wolves and other predators. As humans' needs for help from animals increased, they selected dogs to participate in various helpful tasks. The genetic history of the hunting dog goes back to the Spanish pointer. Even though Brittanys have pointing and retrieving traits, evidence indicates that the Brittany developed not from pointing or retrieving breeds, but rather from a separate line of dogs. The ancient dog and the wolf each had the ability to point and retrieve.

The philosophy of breeding purebred animals varies tremendously from one breeder to another. Some restrictions in breeding include having the ability to use isolation of a gene marker that identifies carrier animals with genetic defects. A breeding challenge is mating dogs that have wanted traits and conformation and exclusion of unwanted genes that carry defects. Obviously, we want to avoid breeding animals that have unwanted genetic factors, including dogs with seizures, or orthopedic, endocrine, dermatological or myriad other health problems. Carrier animals with genetic recessive traits present problems because to the eye such animals appear perfectly normal.

Such animals give breeders handicaps in eliminating unwanted defects before conception. Background checks and information from previous generations are needed to breed healthy animals. Genetic markers detect carrier animals by improving breeding strategies. Unfortunately, to date no genetic markers have been found in the Brittany for detection of unwanted traits before breeding.

Preparation for competition

In breeding, I have selected for the orange roan color pattern. Dogs with this color pattern have foot pads resistant to pad trauma when running on sand, rocky, or volcanic rocky areas. Dogs with orange-and-white-colored hair coats do not have strong feet or pads. Roan-colored dogs seem to consistently have good scenting ability and stamina to run in varying terrains while doing field work.

Preparation to show a dog in competition involves a learning curve. Understanding how to read a dog and how to anticipate that the dog is going to move or break point before it happens is important to championship success. It

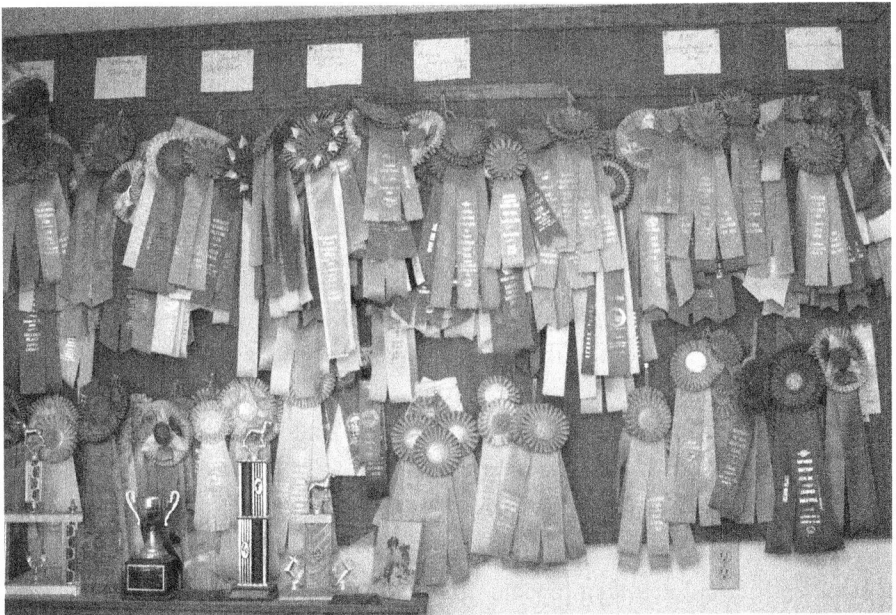

Collection of ribbons in gaining Brittany championships by trialing dogs in the field, gained by the Boy with the Wounded Thumb field trial Brittanys.

225

took me at least five years of competition to effectively learn to properly show a field dog. I was tutored by another handler and trainer in how to direct my dog. I was shown what a competition dog must understand before showing in the field. Most important was maintaining the dog's enthusiasm and desire to please at all times. Gentile teaching mantra was always a training venue, never gruff correction beyond gently showing the dog what was expected. Dogs have excellent memories, and heavy-handed training is often remembered as unpleasant and can lead to poor competition performances years later.

Communication between handler and dog is achieved by eye contact. A handler must use same body language in trials and training periods. To consistently place and win, a handler must know how to read his or her dog and anticipate what the dog will do before moving only under command.

I learned only after years of observation and practice how to train a dog to hold point; when the bird was in the air the dog was trained to immediately stop and not chase. It was given a command by voice or whistle to release and find another bird. This prevents a dog running off under its own command. I initially let a dog learn on its own, as do wolf and coyote pups. For instance, I did not want Luc, one of my early dogs, to chase rabbits, and broke him from doing so by shooting one and then tying it around his neck so he could not loosen it while walking around. When he tired of carrying the rabbit around he no longer wanted to run after one. Most trainers use force of one type or another to train a dog to stop an unwanted behavior. Training a dog to be steady to wing and shot until given the command to go after the bird takes special training techniques.

Max Holland, a local bird dog field trial trainer and owner of Blue Ridge Kennel in Dixon, California, taught me intricacies and finesse used in training a dog to compete in field trialing as a "broke" dog. Max worked with me and gave valuable training advice. I asked him after initial trialing FC Jean-Luc, Luc's son, why certain handlers frequently won and placed dogs while others like me rarely did. I clearly remember his reply: "Know what your dog is going to do before he does it." Wow, what did that mean?

It meant that the most important thing in training a dog is to never take eye contact off him, and watch muscle movements, direction of nose in pointing, eye movement, confidence, and intensity on point in contrast to softness, crouching or sitting. From that moment, I had a life-changing experience in field trialing, and I was on my way to consistently placing with enough wins to stay involved for years.

I emphasized in training for breaking dogs a philosophy allowing them to continue to have freedom to find birds and have enjoyment. It is important for a highly motivated dog to have independence and freedom in what they are doing. Hunting dogs should continue to use their own unique genetic makeup to excel in scenting birds and be aware of different species of wild game. Field trial dogs are trained to compete in a manmade world of unnatural dog desires. It takes special training to achieve placements and championships in field trials and for the dog to remain independent. This fine line of difference in successful training is difficult to explain, and is achieved only by genetic selection and careful training to avoid diminishing desire from a dog while maintaining handler control through which the dog responds to voice or whistle commands.

Field trial circuit

As my experience with Brittanys expanded, I became interested in showing under judgment, which meant participation in organized "field trials." My hunting hobby expanded dramatically when I retired from UC Davis in January 1993. When it came to hunting dog achievement, the line I selected originated from Gianoli's Pat, a superb hunting dog. I hunted with a small group of friends. It took training to compete against other dogs with a set of adhered rules under judgment to achieve recognition. This led to Luc's desirable national recognition.

Luc did well in a non-breed club trials held at Lake Camanche Hunt Club, east of Stockton, California, in the Sierra Nevada foothills. The ribbons earned were conversation pieces because no championship points were earned, and no broke dog stakes were acknowledged by AKC.

I advanced to running Luc under judgment in AKC sanctioned trials. Competing in an AKC or American Field trial required a dog trained to be steady to wing and shot. I was competing in a new game, not bringing meat to the table. The prizes were placement ribbons. Other fulfillment performance standards had to be met to earn placement ribbons, of which blue and red, denoting first and second place, were the most important. The yellow third-place and the white fourth-place ribbons demonstrate that a dog competed well, but in judges' minds is not good enough to earn a blue or red ribbon that carries points toward championship.

As young dogs were added to our field trial circuit string, we more commonly traveled to distant field trial events, which meant staying in a motel or using a sleeping bag on the ground or in a pickup bed. That prompted us to buy a 24-foot gooseneck stock trailer, which we bought at the 4-Star Trailers factory in Oklahoma City. It was functionally built to travel among field trial grounds. The front was converted into living quarters; the middle section, designed as a three-saddle tack area, had room for six dog crates. The rear section had wide swinging entry doors and room for three horses.

After picking up the trailer from the factory, I traveled to Iowa to compete in the Midwest American Brittany Club (ABC) futurity, held 100 miles south of Des Moines. The trailer's living quarters had not yet been built, so I padded the gooseneck area with horse saddle blankets as insulation for my sleeping bag, and I used a small propane camp gas stove to cook meals. On that maiden voyage, I traveled alone. The distance from home to return a month later was 6,000 miles. I stopped every four to six hours to let four dogs out for exercise, and in Oklahoma I purchased two horses. I let the horses out to exercise and eat every 10 to 12 hours. I was fortunate to find places to stable the horses every night on the trip. I would find a place to pull off, usually a truck stop, and I would rest, taking 15-minute naps. I had successful trialing with juvenile bitch "Babe" placing third in the futurity field trial and runner-up bitch in the futurity show, missing dual dog of the show award by one point. Jean-Luc competed in broke dog stakes and had a wonderful all-age run, but was birdless, and did not place.

I began my journey home by traveling to western Iowa to visit relatives in Le Mars. It was the last time I saw my cousin Bud Scholer, who died not long afterward from a heart attack. Bud and I had good summer vacations together when he came to visit us in Minnesota when I was 9 to 11 years old (as described in chapter 6). From Le Mars I traveled to western Minnesota and stabled my horses with my cousin Odell Schaller. After a short visit of three days I was on my way to South Dakota near Rapid City to stay with Dr. Bob and Helen Hanson, good friends who had moved from Davis, California, to the Black Hills area, where Bob practiced human radiology.

Upon my departure on Good Friday morning Bob followed until we came to a fork in the road, where Bob turned north to do professional work at Spearfish, Wyoming. We stopped to say goodbye as I headed south toward Salt Lake City on a two-lane Wyoming state highway. Bob warned me that a lot of people fall asleep on that hypnotically monotonous road. He advised me to stop often and exercise, and get a lot of fresh air, in order to stay awake. Bob said, "Today, we remember Christ dying on the Cross for our salvation. Go with Him accompanying you." That was the last time I saw Bob and Helen, and I vividly remember the trek to expand my capabilities of showing dogs in various parts of the nation. It was Good Friday 1993, and I traveled with the Lord.

I reached western Salt Lake City about 1 a.m. on Saturday, and stayed on property owned by a field trial friend. He previously told me he would not be there when I arrived, but he invited me to use his space to exercise my horses and dogs and to park my trailer and pickup truck. I awoke by 4 a.m. and headed west on I-80. I ate a good brunch at Elko, Nevada. I called Carolyn and told her I would be home for Easter. Another 12 hours of driving remained ahead of me. To drive alone with horses and dogs always was a huge responsibility. The journey was tiring for dogs and horses, and yet they seemed to enjoy traveling. Sitting hour after hour and driving alone took stamina; the danger of falling asleep at the wheel was a constant threat. I never forgot Bob Hanson's advice during each fall trial circuit as I traveled several times from Dixon, California to various trial sites in California, Oklahoma, Texas, Kansas, and Boonville, Arkansas. I usually traveled alone and with the Lord. Country music was always available on the tape deck or radio.

Most trial events were held on weekends. These travel experiences led to meeting special people. Some became friends forever. Field trial people are dedicated dog persons who make sacrifices to go long distances, leaving on Friday evenings, traveling all night to trial grounds, running dogs on Saturday and Sunday, and returning home Sunday night, often arriving just in time to clean up and go to work on Monday morning. At times, a pickup pulling a trailer would break down and require help to fix a broken part, or pull a rig out of mud, snow, or deep gravel. Most trail people were always ready to help another in such need, as I did on several occasions.

Harold Nesham

One man with an unforgettable attitude, ready to help field trial people continue coming or going from an event, was Harold Nesham. I received enormous help from him at Red Rock Field Trial Grounds (BLM land) north of Reno and a bit east of U.S. 395. The day before beginning that trip I had new brake shoes installed on the truck. On Friday, I traveled 170 miles from Dixon to Red Rock Field Trial Grounds.

On Sunday after the trial I left the trial grounds and drove five miles on a dirt and gravel road, heading toward a surfaced county road. One mile from the asphalt road, I suddenly heard a loud *bang* and my truck veered to the right. Because I was traveling at only 10 miles per hour on the rough gravel road, I was able to stop in a shallow ditch within a few seconds. My pickup truck's right front wheel had collapsed. I hitchhiked five miles back to camp to obtain Harold's help. Harold was loading up horses to return home to Sacramento. He brought the horses to rent to persons needing a horse to handle a dog by horseback. He had been a handler for years and when semi-retired bought horses to rent at trials for extra income. He had a loudspeaker on his rig and every morning about 5:30 a.m. would awaken the camp by announcing, "Time to arise, field trialers."

Upon hearing of my plight, Harold immediately stopped what he was doing, detached his pickup, and drove to my rig. He determined that the brake calipers had collapsed and we needed to have the rig brought back to the field trial grounds. We called AAA, and a tow truck hauled my rig back to camp because fixing the pickup alongside the gravel road in a shallow ditch would have been difficult.

With the pickup jacked up in camp, Harold found that the caliper bolts were only finger tight; they probably had not been adequately tightened when the brake job was done the prior Thursday, resulting in the collapse. I needed new calipers to replace the damaged ones. Harold and I drove 20 miles to a parts store, which did not have the needed calipers in stock. We had to wait until Monday morning to get parts from a Ford dealership. By the time we obtained the parts, returned to camp, and installed the new calipers, it was Monday afternoon. I offered to pay Harold for his time; he agreed to accept payment for only half of his time and nothing for staying over a full day to help get me back on the road. What a wonderful man.

Harold always was there to help people in need at the trial grounds, including helping others broken down on the way to or from the grounds. He provided horses for trialers and charged a minimal amount so people could ride horseback while showing their dogs. He had a special horse, a mare called "Mandy," that in my veterinary experiences was a unique equine. She immediately knew when an inexperienced rider was on her, and would accommodate accordingly. She continued to be a wrangler's horse until she was 44 years old. Wow, what a miraculous mare with personality, ability, an equine with the highest IQ I ever encountered. She really talked with her eyes and could carry on a "conversation" with eye-to-eye contact.

Harold unfortunately received little recognition despite all that he did. After his death no members of any dog club wrote a note in his memory. He was a World War II military veteran, and his funeral arranged by relatives was held at the Sacramento Valley National Cemetery near Dixon. I attended his funeral, and I am confident that the many people whom he helped never will forget him.

I continued to participate in field trials until I turned 80 years old, when due to back problems, I gave up riding my horse; I still trained dogs, although with less intensity. I continued to hunt pheasants at Hastings Island Hunting Preserve, 25 miles south of Dixon. Due to physical handicaps I was able to hunt only from field roads but was still able to see my dogs hunt, which enabled me to stay involved with them.

Veterinary care at trials

At trials, it was not uncommon for a horse or dog owner to approach with questions about an ill animal, many of which needed veterinary attention. I diagnosed and treated literally hundreds of animals in the field while attending trials over 25 to 30 years of trialing. In addition to answering questions about ill animals, I frequently discussed breeding strategies. The need for diagnosis and care of animals with chronic problems often of genetic origin was a recurrent topic. Many performance problems in field trialing and hunting were due to training faults induced by humans.

Dogs that are bred to run swiftly through all types of ground cover looking for game are at high risk to inhale mature plant awns that have tiny barbs providing a nidus for bacterial entry as inhaled or puncture wounds. Barbs allow the awn to latch onto an animal and then be transported to a new site to take root. The western United States and north central Canada fescue range grass plants of several different species have barbed awns. These fescue grasses mature in southern portions in April and in the northern section in late September. Summer is the most dangerous time to train a dog in high-risk areas. The awn may migrate through the lung or thoracic cavity and exit as an abscess on the body wall exterior surface, or it may migrate to thoracic organs, including the heart, causing severe pericarditis, or to the back and lodge in a sub-vertebral or vertebral space. A foxtail may remain embedded in a lung. In many cases death results when migration does not allow escape of abscessed pus. The thoracic spaces may fill with enormous quantities of blood, lymphatic fluid, and exudate containing various types of bacteria. The saga of migration varies tremendously in each affected dog.

On one evening at the Brittany Nationals at Blue Mountain Wildlife Demonstration Area near Booneville, Arkansas, I was asked to examine four dogs on the grounds. All of these dogs were qualified to run in the Nationals within a day or two. Each of these four dogs had similar history of running during summer camp training in terrain where cheat grass awns were plentiful. All had been coughing, and their enthusiasm for running was sharply diminished. In each case I diagnosed inhaled cheat grass or an inhaled foreign body. I indicated that three of the four needed immediate veterinary attention, which they received the next day. Two underwent an emergency thoracotomy to drain pus and were placed on antibiotics. The third was placed on broad-spectrum antibiotics and recovered with long-term medication. The fourth dog stayed on the grounds, was placed on broad-spectrum antibiotics, and ran in the Nationals two days later. She later had recurrence and also had a thoracotomy. This dog, DC/AFC Pokie Dot, became a Hall of Fame recipient.

Our bitch, Breton's Babe Ain't She Sweet, coughed after training in early May. She had inhaled a foxtail plant awn. Coughing stopped in a few hours, giving the impression the object had been eliminated. Five days later, though, she developed a fever and depression. X-ray and ultrasound examination revealed she had a left cardiac lung lobe abscess, obviously from the foreign body. She was placed on a regimen of antibiotics for four weeks and remained well for about two months, when symptoms recurred and X-rays showed renewed abscessation of the left lung that extended beyond the cardiac lobe.

Thoracic surgeons suggested thoracotomy with total removal of the left lung. If she survived the procedure, she no longer would have lung capacity for field trials. With that likely outcome, I placed her on daily antibiotics, which I never stopped the rest of her life. She developed a severe neurological disorder at age 13 as an AFC (amateur field trial champion) and MH (master hunter), and retained strong desire to hunt until her death in her 13th year. Foreign bodies can be removed successfully by endoscopic approach before abscessation occurs. Recovery is such cases in quick and uneventful. Unfortunately quick cessation of coughing after inhalation gives a false sense of security that the object has been coughed out. If such coughing is ignored for a day, abscessation from accompanying bacteria occurs.

Dog club membership

My association with the Northern California Brittany Club (NCBC) began in early 1970. The club had been organized in 1954 as an affiliate of the parent national organization, the American Brittany Club (ABC), which was established in the early 1930s. NCBC holds two field trials each year and a specialty conformation show once a year. A Fun Days event is held the last weekend of July every year. This activity brings in new members and encourages dog lovers of other breeds to attend by holding educational seminars for dog owners of all hunting breeds. I was awarded a huge honor by being voted to receive NCBC Lifetime Membership. This honor was one of the finest awards I have received in my hobby career.

I served on the board of directors of the parent club, ABC, for 15 years. I also served as chair of the Genetics and Health Aspects Committee and member of subcommittees. I wrote several health and genetic reports for publication in the ABC magazine, and I conducted a health questionnaire in 1976 with added information about the breed's qualities and health issues. I was inducted into the ABC Hall of Fame, another special recognition connected to my hobby of field trialing and breeding high-quality dogs. In 2007, I additionally was inducted into the Brittany Field Trial Hall of Fame at the Bird Dog Hall of Fame in Grand Junction, Tennessee. A record of that award is placed in the Hall of Fame Museum. This is an amazing museum about bird dogs of all breeds and persons dedicated to improve the sport.

Mr. Larry Hagedorn, the President of the Southern Kansas Brittany Club, asked me to help initiate a memorial for a deceased member of their club, Captain Marvin D. Nelson Jr. A memorial fund was created at UC Davis to provide money for study of genetic diseases in the Brittany. That resulted in establishment of a Brittany DNA library, samples from which contributed to study of genetic diversity in the Brittany. The resulting knowledge has potential to improve genetic information to strengthen the breed and instigate research to discover gene markers to help eliminate carrier animals.

Accolades

I was fortunate to have "Rex," the family German shepherd, at my side when I nearly accidentally lost my right thumb at age 5. This terrorizing moment was the most impressive life-changing event in my life. From an early age, I saw beauty and purpose in all types of animals, and had a deep interest in all of God's creatures.

I was attracted to birds of all types and the color of their eggs and structure of their nests fascinated me. Observation of pigeons, doves and domesticated chickens brought great satisfaction. Farm animals always have been of interest to me, with horses highest on the list, while my mule "Derby" was tops of all four-legged hoofed animals. I especially revere a gentle milking shorthorn small cow, "Red," because she was the cow I learned to hand milk at a young age. When I was especially tired at evening milking time, I would lie in hay in the manger in front of Red and go to sleep as she ate hay around me.

Cats have had a special soft spot in my life. I marvel at their ability to secretly communicate and show concern and affection in ways unknown to other species. Winston Churchill, who revered animals, said that "cats look down on us," but he did not observe inner feline traits. Our cat "Bob," a Manx breed born with a bobbed tail like many Brittanys, is a working cat. She seems to soothe my anxieties about daily problems, and during such times is near or on my lap or asleep at the foot of the bed.

All of the many Brittany dogs whelped, owned, raised, trained, and competed under the Breton Kennels name were special. These dogs intrigued me about the origin of the breed and their unique genetic makeup, as well as their abilities to perform in a variety of situations. They have brought joy and inspiration to my life.

God provided the Boy With the Wounded Thumb dreams to professionally be with all His creatures. He gave me the desire to share knowledge with clients, friends, and family, and enjoy dogs, horses and mules, and my favorite hobbies of hunting wild game and showing dogs in the field. The dream of being a veterinarian fulfilled a philosophy I shared with students while teaching at UC Davis "to live a balanced triad." I suggested this was an axiom on a successful professional life if one employed a balance with faith in God (as chapter 14 describes). I was blessed to fulfill my childhood dream about veterinary care. My discoveries of causes of some forms of cancers and development of treatment and prevention programs as the originator of veterinary cancer medicine became frosting on the cake of my life. *One Medicine War on Cancer,* focuses on that basic cancer research and the emergence and evolution of veterinary cancer medicine.

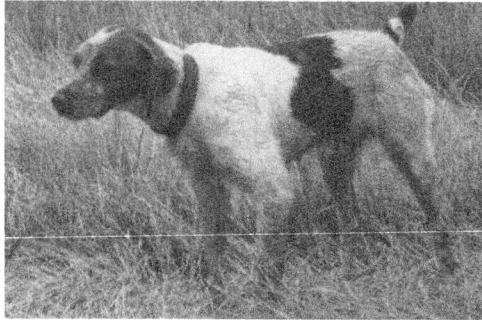

FC Jean-Luc Le Breton (AKC SF0464477), "Jean-Luc"

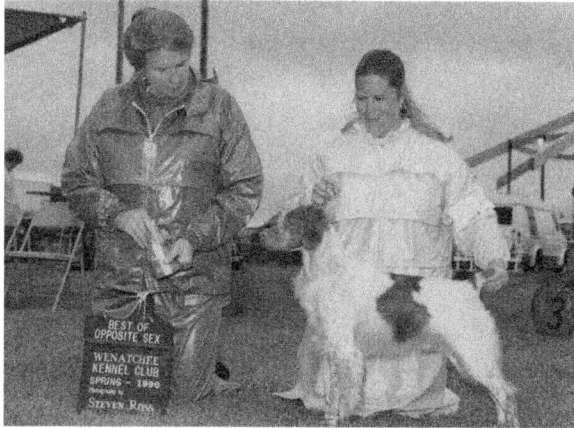

Show placement

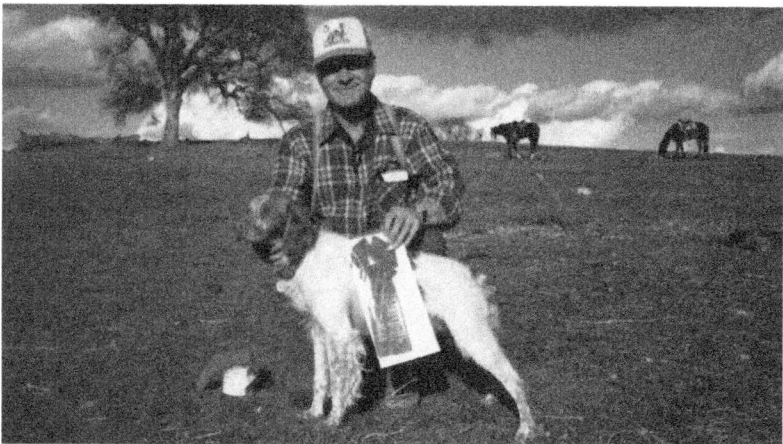

1st adult dog field placement, 2nd place, Santa Nella, California

APPENDIX

The Genetic Legacy of Breton Kennels, Dixon, California

After I joined the Northern California Brittany Club in 1970, I was encouraged to show my Brittany Luc Le Breton SH (AKC-SD600625), known as "Luc," under judgment in field trial competition. I entered a trail held at the Grizzly Island field trial grounds, surrounded by marshland 10 miles south of Suisun, California.

Luc was much superior to most dogs entered as a hunting dog, and none of the others had bayed wild hogs. He was entered in the "gun dog" category, in which he had to hold point while a gunner came to shoot a pen-raised bird, a chucker. I was required to push the bird with my foot to prompt it to fly. The rules call for a dog to be steady to wing and shoot. As a self-taught hunting dog, Luc had no training to wait until being sent to retrieve. As soon as the bird had been shot and was on the ground, Luc had it and retrieved beautifully to hand. He was disqualified, though, because he broke on the shot. He held point beautifully until the shot was fired. Wham, he was off for retrieve. He was a superb retriever for wild bird hunting in the Nevada desert, California flat or hilly country blind retrieves, where he was not able to see the bird fall. He swam over fast-moving streams, lakes, or canals to retrieve a bird to hand. In certain conditions he would retrieve two birds one after the other when two or more were shot (a double-kill) at one time. Luc and I were bonded and rarely separated except when I was traveling or at work. He often went with me on veterinary calls or other places, and he would stay in the car or truck, not exiting unless asked.

While hunting at Hastings Island Hunting Preserve in Rio Vista, I met Lynn and Jack Guzman. They were dedicated Brittany owners of two bitches who were impressed with Luc's ability to hold point forever and then to go, if necessary, several hundred yards to make a retrieve. We mutually decided to mate one of their bitches, Jodi, to Luc.

Jacklyn's Princess Jodi (AKC SD489653), "Jodi"

Jodi was a white-and-orange-colored Brittany bitch that was a hunting companion. The mating with Luc resulted in birth of eight beautiful pups. Four were orange and roan, and four were orange and white. We accepted two male pups from the litter, both colored orange roan. We kept one, Jean-Luc Le Breton, and the other, Pat, became the hunting dog and pet for Dr. Bill Frost, the stepson of my colleague Dr. John Hughes. About that time I began to think of breeding with my own Breton Kennels not as a commercial enterprise, but rather as a means to approach the process of breeding selections from a scientific basis, with the intention of making improvements in the genetics of the breed.

Jean-Luc Le Breton, a special hunting dog, was my first dog to be trained to compete as a broke dog under judgment. His field showing was competing in horseback-handled stakes in an event known as "open all age." He was nationally recognized for desire, ground speed, and ranging to the extent of the course. Jean-Luc was a phenomenal versatile hunter, like his sire, Luc, and great-grand sire, Gianoli's Pat. Jean-Luc was an exceptional all-around dog that would adapt to hunting different game bird species under different environmental conditions. He was an eye opener to watch running in field trials, never flat, always ready to run with utmost enthusiasm. He would go to the limits of the course to find game, which might be miles away under competition judgment.

He was in contention for placement at the National All Age Championship in Booneville, Arkansas, in 1997 with three flawless quail covey finds and a fourth find with great style. The brace mate handler came galloping as fast as he could during Jean-Luc's find to stop his dog who he knew would not honor. He yelled at the top of his voice "whoa, whoa, whoa!" to no avail to stop his dog. As the handler got close on horseback to Jean-Luc, he lost intensity and sat, in response to thinking he had done something wrong. This movement resulted in the judge's decision to have the dog collared. The dog moved and was out of competition. The command by the judge to "Pick up your dog" means an error or movement was committed, eliminating the dog for placement consideration. A year later when one of the judges and I rode by the spot where that happened, he told me, "this is where you lost the National Championship with Jean-Luc last year." Wow, he came so close and yet because of one flaw he did not win the American Brittany Club (ABC) All Age National Championship. I never again had a dog that was close to placing or winning at the All Age Nationals.

Jean-Luc, who was a beautiful orange roan in color, achieved show points but did not finish as a show champion. In the show circuit in which he participated few judges placed roan-colored dogs. Many did not know the color was standard. Jean-Luc, a dog that could never be replaced, lived 15 years. He was a one-of-a-kind Brittany that almost won the Nationals and was never equaled as an all-age national contester or as a versatile hunting dog that bayed wild hogs.

Jean-Luc was one of the few, if any other dogs, to compete in all three Brittany futurities. The ABC futurities are events that showcase Brittany breeders and recognize their dogs that show promise as representative of the best genetic traits of the breed. The Eastern part was held in Medford, New Jersey, at the New England Setter Club, the Central in Southern Illinois in snow- and sleet-covered terrain, and the Western in Eastern Washington state. Jean-Luc competed in trials in Upstate New York, New Jersey, Iowa, Missouri, Arkansas, Kansas, Oklahoma, Texas, Arizona, California, Oregon, Idaho, and Washington. People who saw him compete never forgot the high standard he set. He traveled 30,000 miles by plane, covering a good portion of the United States, and another 30,000 miles by road.

The genetic uniqueness of Luc and Jean-Luc was largely due to inheritance from Gianoli Pat, the ancestor unknown except to Al Gianoli's close hunting friends. Pat was the foundation sire of the Breton Kennels line. He epitomized boldness, a grievously ignored American Brittany trait. He bestowed a regal personality that is evident in a portrait hanging in our home.

The vocabulary of dog trials

Participation in dog trial competitions requires familiarity with specific terms and their abbreviations.

AFC: Amateur Field Trial Champion title
AKC: American Kennel Club
CH: Champion
DC: Dual Champion
FC: Field Champion
GC: Grand Show Champion
HOF: Hall of Fame
NAFC: National Amateur Field Champion
NFC: National Field Champion
JH, SH, MH: Junior, Senior, Master Hunter

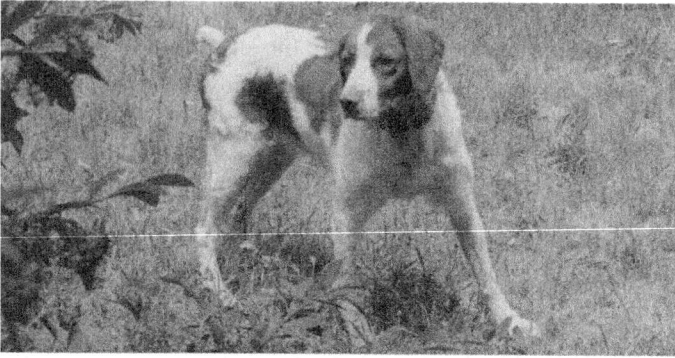

AFC Breton's Babe Ain't She Sweet MH (AKC SM835797/05), "Babe"

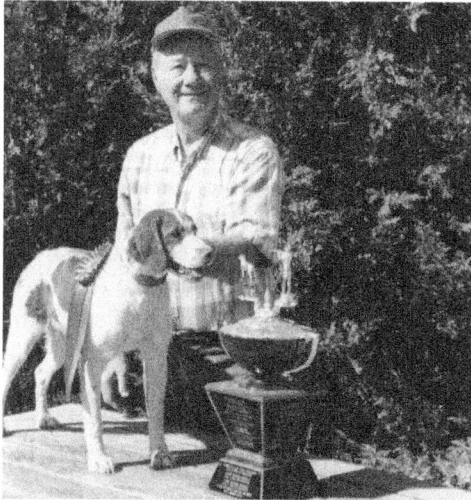

1st place with Amateur Gun Dog trophy, Ionia, Michigan

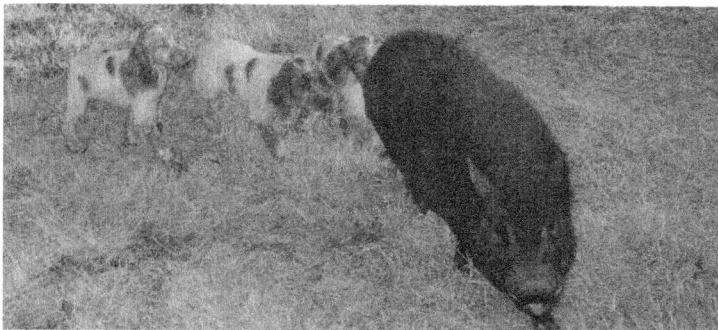

Training pups to hunt wild hogs chasing a pet pig

Babe was whelped in Idaho at Lobo's Kennel, owned by well-known Brittany breeders Mr. and Mrs. Bob Lanham. Babe was sired by FC/AFC Lobo's Blazing Candy Man out of DC Lobo's Sugar Babe. She was the granddaughter of NFC and Hall of Fame Bean's Blaze. Babe was a replacement for a female pup I had purchased a year earlier, Breton's Flamme, who had a mild condition of hip dysplasia diagnosed at 11 months with radiographs. Flamme was spayed and sold because her genetic connection with hip dysplasia diminished her usefulness as a breeding bitch. She was purchased by retired Air Force Colonel West, an upland game hunter of most wild bird species found in North America. Flamme never developed clinical signs of hip dysplasia, hunted five months a year until she was 14 years old, and died at the age of 15.

Babe became an outstanding bird dog and pointed with style that few Brittanys could emulate. Babe had a wonderful personality and overall was a needed addition to our kennel. Her warm attitude is displayed in a portrait hanging in our home. She whelped three litters, most of the pups of which became good bird dogs. We never kept a pup for adding to the Breton Kennels gene pool. The pups we evaluated as young dogs did not fit into our breeding program. We purchased another female to mate with Jean-Luc from one of dog trainer Dave Walker's clients who lived in the state of Washington.

Jewelry X-Press (AKC SM94506104), "Jewel"

I purchased Jewel to mate with Jean-Luc in order to perpetuate his outstanding performance and add to the Breton Kennels gene pool. Jewel was a bit shy and soft because Dave Walker had attempted to train her for field trials but found that her personality was not suitable for field trialing. We determined that her outstanding pedigree outweighed any concerns about personality traits.

Jewel was two years old and sired by NFC, FC, AFC Bean's Blaze Hall of Fame, out of Ron's Ban-Dee Amber Lace. Her pedigree indicated she would be a wonderful female to perpetuate wanted hunting traits by mating to Jean-Luc. We kept a male orange roan, Jean-Luc Picard, "Captain" from the first and only litter whelped by Jewel, who developed a uterine infection, leading to her being spayed. We sold Jewel to a wonderful pet/hunting home, where she lived for 14 years as a pet and hunting dog. She was euthanized as she neared old age death, and buried in the Field of Dreams, a special place for burial known only to a few people.

Captain was an outstanding hunting and field trial dog, soft like his dam, and needed careful training. Captain sired a few litters, never hunted wild hogs, and never was used as previous Breton Kennels dogs as a versatile hunting dog. Captain died in 2012 at age 16.

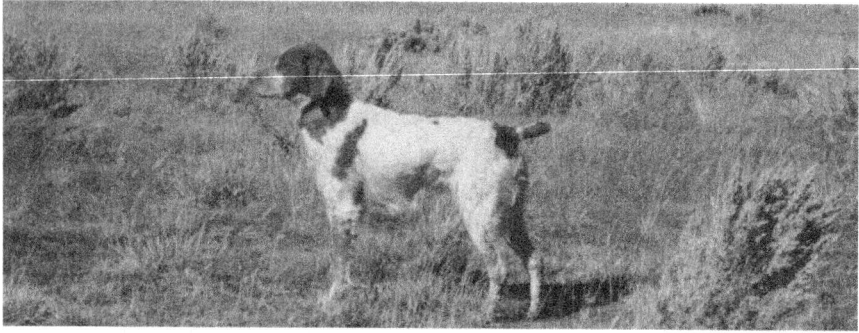

FC Breton's Jean-Luc Picard (AKC SN34962803), "Captain" pointing, chukar Red Rock Trial Grounds, Reno, Nevada.

Lady Ruffles Little Brit (AKC SE665908), "Brit"

Brit, an orange-and-white bitch with sound genetic background, was owned by Elizabeth Carlson. She was a pet and never was used as a hunting dog. The mating with Jean-Luc produced eight pups. Most were exceptional bird dogs. Lisa Lengtat purchased one roan male, Russ, as a gift for her husband, Tom, who wanted a hunting dog. This purchase developed into a lifelong friendship with Tom and Lisa. I went on several superb California valley quail hunting outings with Tom at his aunt and uncle's ranch near Coalinga, California. Quail were extremely numerous and dogs had no problem in pointing coveys.

Tom and Lisa vacationed in Hawaii when Russ was 5 years old. They left Russ in my care. As I prepared to take Russ and my three dogs for exercise, I tied them to the all-terrain vehicle for roading exercise. Before I left, I was interrupted for a five-minute phone call, while Russ remained in the kennel. When I went to fetch Russ in the kennel run, I found him hanging from a long bolt, in which his lead had become tangled. He was unconscious, and my attempts using mouth-to-mouth resuscitation and CPR failed to revive him. He was dead, and I had no contact number to reach Tom and Lisa in Hawaii. Russ became a member in the Field of Dreams, a permanent resting place. It was an emotional moment when Tom and Lisa learned what had happened to Russ. I removed the long bolt to prevent another dog from hanging itself, which never happened again.

From this litter, my colleague Dr. John Hughes acquired Fergie, an orange and white bitch puppy. John obtained this dog as he was getting older and did less hunting, although Fergie was a wonderful companion and went along on cattle roundups and loved to run alongside John while he was riding horses in mountain terrain. She had the run of the house and would always be at the front door to greet guests, as I often experienced. I will never forget the warm greetings of this fine Brittany when the front door was opened. We acquired three pups – a bitch named CO-CO, a male named Timbre, and another female named Vallee Gold from this litter.

Vallee Gold was an outstanding competitor in hunting and the field. She would hold point for 15 minutes or longer if the circumstances called for her to stay. Unfortunately, Vallee developed a severe uterine infection and had to be spayed. I gave her to an older couple who loved to hunt, and Vallee became a hunting companion. When she was 15 years old, she was euthanized for severe geriatric problems and became another member in the Field of Dreams.

Timber did not make it as a trial dog. He too was a wonderful hunting dog and had all the attributes to please any dedicated hunter. I sold Timbre to restaurateurs in Southern California, Elisia and Salvitori Scardonos, as their hunting dog. Unfortunately, "Tim" developed advanced cancer at 8 years of age and had to be euthanized.

CO-CO was a fine orange roan bitch sired by FC Jean-Luc Le Breton out of Little Brit's. Her dam was Lady Ruffles of Davis sired by FC Del Oro's Mini Timber and great grand sire DC Timberex. A former student and colleague of mine, Professor Gary Carlson, his wife, Ann, and their children, Christie, Elizabeth, and Tom, were all involved in raising Little Brit's pups. Pups from the mating of Jean-Luc and Little Brit were socialized with people and dogs. Puppy environment is important, with good care and constant handling to help prepare them for excellence adult performance.

CO-CO became the extension of the gene pool from Gianoli's Pat. She was tireless in performance and all activities. She exemplified the special traits from her ancestors. CO-CO was bold as she was selected to be, slivering

243

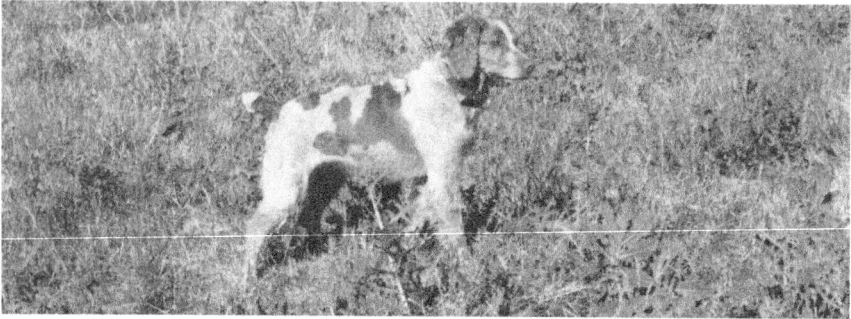

FC/AFC Breton's Cognac (AKC SM9864465/01), "CO-CO" holding point on a pheasant at Suisun Marsh, California.

through tall, thick tules just like a Labrador retriever to find game. She held point for many minutes and loved to retrieve, swam considerable distances, and maneuvered through marshes and other obstacles to fetch a bird and bring it back to hand.

CO-CO's sweet personality along with her hunting attributes brought a dimension to the Breton Kennels that would last forever; she was a natural pointer, natural backer, and a natural retriever. She was a complete hunting dog that exemplified Brittany hunting ability par excellence. But at 8 years of age she developed a rapidly spreading extensive cancer, a rare form of carcinomatosis that spread to most tissues of her body. CO-CO's portrait hangs in our living room. Her gentleness is obvious as expressed with a cocked head, as if he had been spoken to and was replying "what can I do for you?" CO-CO was mated once by frozen semen insemination with a nationally known dog, Tyrone.

ANFC/FC/AFC Rebel's Tough Is Tyrone (AKC SN08890802), "Tyrone"

Tyrone was an orange roan dog from Kansas that Dr. Fran Savage, DVM, and her father, Marvin D. Nelson Jr., owned. Tyrone was tough as nails and sired four pups: three males and one female. All pups were orange roan as were Tyrone and CO-CO. We kept a male named "Sun" and sold the others. Rebel's Tough is Tyrone was a superb bird dog and tireless competitor. He was campaigned by trainer and handler Jimmie John. Fran and two of her three sons were killed in a car accident on the way from Nebraska to show NFC/FC/

AFC Tequila's Joker near Minneapolis. After the car accident tragedy, Tyrone was placed with her father, co-owner, Capt. Marvin D. Nelson Jr. Tyrone, unfortunately escaped from the backyard and was killed on a busy street. Tyrone was not aware that cars are lethal weapons.

FC/AFC Breton's Co-Dee lived with Laurie and Steve Ralph in Minnesota. This dog did not make it on the trial circuit running under Jimmie John but did well when handled with owner Steve Ralph, who finished him as FC/AFC. Steve had once indicated to me he was the best hunting dog in his kennel. The other male, Breton's Jean-Luc Pierre, was purchased by Professor James Cullor, DVM, and his wife Mary. The dog, nicknamed "Petie," became a hunting dog and housedog. Petie was gentle like his dam and litter mates. Dr. Cullor had owned Brittanys since his days as a youngster hunting in Kansas; he considered Petie the best hunting dog he had owned.

The female went to a home in Nevada. She showed enormous potential and great desire as a young dog, when she already would point and find game. She became lost shortly while hunting in the desert, however, and was never found.

Sun, who we kept, was one of the finest Brittanys every whelped, which tied together a genetic composition hard if ever possible to repeat. Wow, what a dog. Sun was similar to his grandfather Jean-Luc, and in other ways even more like his great grandfather Luc. His sire, Tyrone, was an extremely bold dog, as were other males on CO-CO's side. There are few Brittanys with noticeable hunting boldness like this line of Brittany even as observed in other breeds, like that found in Chesapeake retrievers or German Shorthair Pointers.

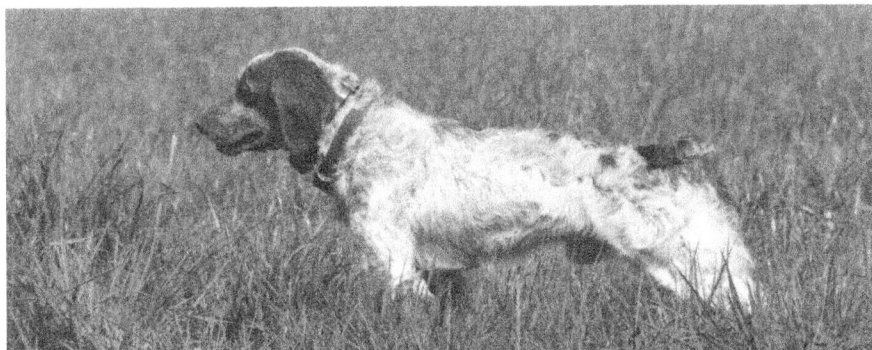

FC Breton's Soleil De Midi (AKC SN65622604), "Sun."

I would classify Sun as a confident, bold dog, yet with a loving personality – the combination of this line, all work in the field, and a loving companion at home with people or other dogs.

Breton's Mon Petit Sourire (AKC SR02965304), "Petit"

Petit was purchased from a kennel in Georgia. She was out of Royal Ruthless by FC/AFC Hi Scor Jac D'Ruffian HOF. She always had a small loving smile, which led to her name Mon Petit Sourire (my little smile). She was a staunch pointing dog with great desire to run. She was never fully trained for field trialing, but was always eager to hunt, and enjoyed association with humans and dogs.

Petit was mated with Sun, resulting in whelping of six pups: two females and four males. They were fine bird dogs, three of which were initially raised to participate in competition. A male, Breton's Run Until I'm Done (Slash), was owned by our adopted family members Mari-Ann and Rick Green, daughter Chondra, and son Kevin. This pup showed as much all-age potential and desire to run in spectacular fashion to the extent of the course as any pup ever whelped at Breton Kennels. He was trained as a field trial dog, but unexpectedly had a severe grand mal seizure, then shortly after that a second near-fatal seizure, and was euthanized. This was the second experience I had with canine epilepsy in dogs whelped in my kennel. Both were whelped from bitches I had purchased as puppies from famous field trial stock. This pup and AFC Breton's Babe Ain't She Sweet MH genetically came out of the Pacific Northwest.

Breton's Monsieur Bert (AKC SR269553206)

Breton's Monsieur Bert was a shorter running dog that was easy to train. We co-owned Bert with our good friend, Chris Zink. Radiographically his hips were rated with mild dysplasia, and we decided to sell him to a good hunting-pet home. He too was a fine bird dog and one with considerable potential. Bert's new home consisted of an acre backyard with a doggie door through which he could go in and out of the house as he desired. He became a good hunting companion and pet for a wonderful family.

Breton's Myever Sol Corbin (AKC SR26953205)

We co-owned Breton's Myever Sol Corbin with Walt and Judy Pryon. Corbin never made it in field trialing, probably due to inconsistent training that lacked focus. He was a beautiful Brittany with excellent conformation.

FC/AFC Texas Crisscross (AKC SN501601), "Criss"

Criss was owned by Kimberly Ramage. Criss mated with Petit, which brought together outstanding pedigree championship lines – on the sire's side, FC/AFC Scipio Spinks, DC Scipio's Little Chick HOF, and on the dam's side FC/AFC Hi-Score Jac D Ruffian HOF, DC/AFC Whiz Kid and NFC, FC/AFC Bean's Blaze HOF.

Breton's Little Texas Smile (AKC), "Gabe"

This mating resulted in desirable bird dogs and development of friendships with several wonderful people. Breton's Little Texas Smile "Gabe" was purchased by Kyle Tetlow, with whom we developed a family friendship. Gabe became a complete package hunting dog. Three of five males in the litter had one undescended testicle, a conformation defect. Gabe was neutered by vasectomy, which allowed the dog to maintain male vigor. My philosophy in selling pups was to remain in close contact with owners of purchased pups. Doing so helped me gain genetic defect information and insight about which breedings warranted repeating.

Breton's Crisscross Sierra (AKC SR491144009), "Sage"

Skip Bickett purchased a female pup that, like her brother, was a complete hunting dog exposed mostly to wild chukar, quail, and pheasant hunting.

Lou Schmitd bought "Jacko," a male pup that became a dedicated hunting companion. Jacko suddenly developed a health problem that was never diagnosed. The condition resulted in kidney failure, and despite heroic medical efforts he died. After his admission to the UC Davis Veterinary Hospital, tests revealed he had developed a blood clotting disorder, von Willebrand's disease. This condition apparently was unrelated to the undiagnosed malady that led to death.

James McCann purchased Charlie Paw (SR49114007), a male that became a fine upland game grouse hunting dog in the Fairbanks, Alaska, region. Charlie pointed and retrieved at an early age, hunted in snow, and was superb at retrieving downed grouse buried in snow.

Sammie (SR491144001), a female, was purchased by Ann Carlson for her husband Professor Gary Carlson. Sammie is a beautiful orange-and-white female pup. She is a good pheasant dog and pet. All of the Carlson dogs were well cared for and excellent household companions.

Tubby, owned by Robert and Joan Donnell, was sired by FC Noble Rocket (AKC SE595540) out of FC Chikamin's Zezebel. She was bred and whelped at Dave Walker's kennel in Idaho. The Donnells indicated that as a young pup, Tubby would climb over a 6-foot kennel fence and escape. She initially was an overweight pup, which is why she was named "Tubby." She later became a well-conditioned thin bitch and was never overweight as an adult.

Noble Rocket, an excellent field champion, had a trialing ending accident as a young dog. While competing in rocky, mountainous terrain, Rocket ran through a drainage creek and was found wedged between rocks with a severely comminuted fracture of the front leg humerus bone – meaning that it was shattered into several pieces. The fracture was so severe that a veterinarian

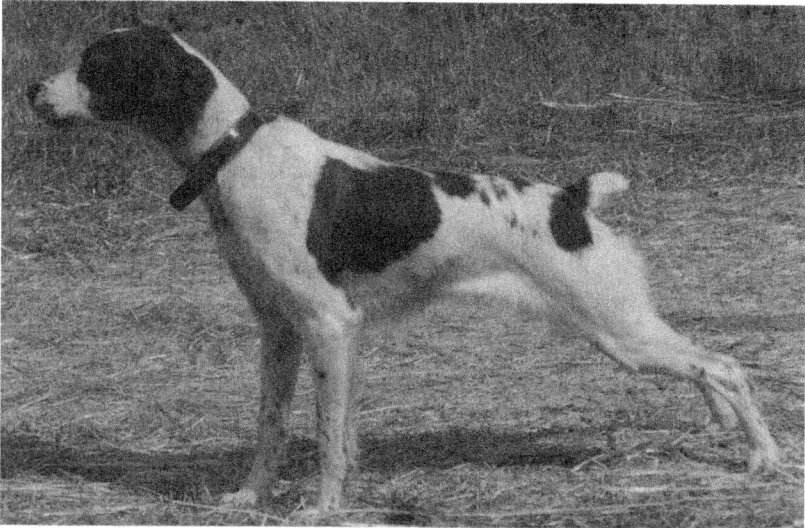

DC/AFC Chikamin's Tub O'Gold (AKC SN426177/02), "Tubby."

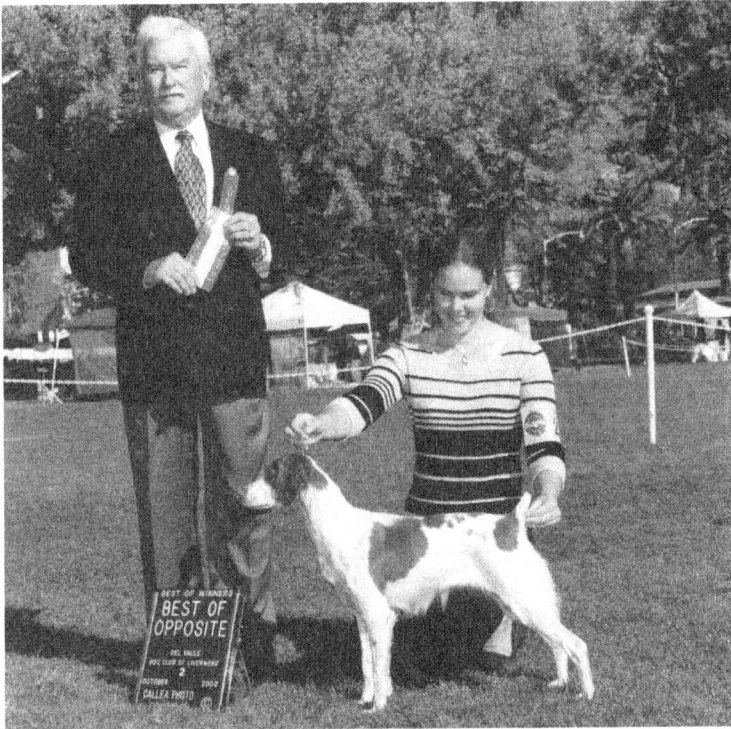

*"Tubby" in show win / best of winners, before she became a dual
champion, shown here with Jessica Carlson.*

determined on initial examination that the leg must be amputated. He would
never recover the ability to run again as a three-legged dog, but lived to sire
Tubby. He was a brother of NFC/FC Beans Blaze HOF and as a young dog
showed equal bird dog promise. Tubby proved to be an excellent offspring.

Zezebel earned her FC but was shown in the field infrequently. When
Tubby's litter reached juvenile status, Robert Donnell had a severe neurological
malady that led to selling Tubby at 15 months of age, with one puppy point
toward championship. Tubby immediately showed field promise and, with me
handling her, earned her derby points and at two years of age became a field
champion (FC).

She would tirelessly run to the extent of the course and often would be
hundreds of yards to the front. Tubby ran a derby event in the Mojave Desert
near California City, and at one point could not be found. She had run several

hundred yards in front the entire time. I circled and circled the course and then another brace was run, which meant others expert brace competitors and judges could be on course. About an hour later, Steve Cosgrave was leaving the grounds pulling a horse trailer attached to his pickup camper rig at a junction a mile or so from the camp. He stopped and asked what I was doing that far from camp, and when I told him about losing Tubby, he immediately stopped, saddled his horse, and began looking with me for the dog. In 15 to 30 minutes, an AKC representative passed on a dirt desert road on the way to the trial. He found Tubby 5 miles from the course. He recognized the she was a Brittany, called her, and she came directly to him. He brought her back to camp. This was the only time she was lost, even in mountainous terrain and seen by my scout a mile or more from the course of trial. After becoming lost that one day in the Mojave Desert, she always sensed my location and would find me.

People who saw Tubby run never forgot her tremendous desire to be in front, whether the ground was covered with cold, wet snow or if the temperature was 90 degrees. She was never flat and always ran with eagerness and zeal. She earned her FC at 2 years of age, and finally at 8 years became an AFC. There were fewer entries in Brittany Amateur All-Age stakes (the class showing extreme independence), meaning it was difficult to win a needed three-point major. American Brittany Club requires a three-point major in a Brittany Club sponsored trial to finish as a field champion.

She placed runner-up in the one-hour ABC Chukar Championship at milepost 9 in Idaho. This was a mountainous course that allowed a spectacular run in a fashion always focused to the front, close to a mile ahead. She pointed two different coveys of chucker and finished going away at least a quarter mile ahead. The brace mate won the chucker championship with a single chucker find, birdless non-productive find at the hour finish. It appeared he was out of energy and did not run further. The winner was improperly placed due to the judge's bias. Judges' decisions at times make no sense, and on this event they missed the winning dog big time.

Tubby loved to be picked up after finishing a huge run and enjoyed riding on the saddle in front. She seemed to exhibit a canine joy during these rides, often a mile or more back to camp. Tubby also loved to travel by riding on the front seat of my pickup truck or snuggling up in the back seat area. She also enjoyed sleeping at the foot of my bed on field trial outings.

Her AFC Championship was achieved in Texas two weeks before whelping six pups on November 26, 2005, at 8 years, 8 months and 18 days of age. When she won AFC, she ran a spectacular all-age race. She was an amazing bitch that gave me continuous sense of satisfaction and high level of confidence as an amateur handler. I never felt we were a lesser quality entry, whether we competed against nationally recognized all-age American Field Champions like English pointers, setters, top-notch all-age German shorthairs, wirehaired pointers, red setters, vizslas, or any other bird dog pointing breed. It was a huge pleasure to show her in the field. I express thankfulness to the Donnells for selling her and for being shown by accomplished dog handler and breeder Jessica Carlson to a show championship (CH) and a dual champion (DC) title.

Tubby was first shown in conformation at 6 years of age and quickly finished CH. She was a natural with a wonderful gait and desire to show to the judge. She loved to perform in conformation and in field competition. Tubby was Jessica's first dual champion, and Jessica went on to finish many DCs, totaling 31 by July 2016. Jessica became a known amateur field handler. Tubby added genes to Breton Kennels in new dimensions that greatly improved genetic lines.

Introduction of Jessica to field trialing is a fond memory. She started as a youngster handling show dogs and became an intelligent handler and amateur trainer. She contributed enormously to ABC events and was editor of the 2012 *Book of the American Brittany: 1990–2010 Edition*. Jessica personally signed a copy for me in which she wrote, "To Gordon: Thank you for your years as a mentor and a friend – it's largely thanks to you that I got to know field trials and the Dual Brittany." – Jessica Carlson.

These words of sincere thanks will live in my heart forever. Jessica is a talented person who has an in-depth compassion for positive thinking and never forgetting how she came to be a writer, artist, conformation handler, and field trailer. I feel honored to have been a part of her accomplishments. She is a true friend and epitomizes American Brittany Club leadership and the goal of bettering the breed.

Tubby was bred three times, the first two by frozen semen artificial insemination – first to "Sparky" and the second time to "Hank" – and then inadvertently to "Captain."

ANFC/FC/AFC Jim De Bob's Sparks A Dan D HOF (AKC SF701149), "Sparky"

The litter sired by Sparky and Tubby consisted of five pups: one female and four males. Steve Ralph purchased the female, who in summer camp training in Montana as a young derby dog inhaled a foreign body – a cheatgrass awn (bristle) that caused acute sudden pneumonia and death. Barbed plant awns carry a variety of bacteria that produce severe inflammation and abscessation when lodged in the lung or other tissues of the body. A male owned by Bernie Crain escaped from the kennel and was killed by a car. A male called Sparky, owned by Mary and Jim Crawford, did well as a field and show dog. Mr. and Mrs. Barry Koepke purchased a male that was neutered for medical reasons. He was entered in field competition, but never earned an FC designation. I kept a male, Cowboy, who had a big run but was not a good bird dog. I sold him to a hunting home. He escaped from that kennel and was in an automobile accident in which he sustained a severely comminuted fractured leg that was amputated. He remained as a kennel pet. Field trial trained big running dogs are at high risk for death by motor vehicles.

FC/AFC Hi Scor Jac D'Ruffian HOF (AKC SM799080), "Hank"

Tubby's frozen semen mating with Hank produced a litter of two males and three females: "Runner," "Page," and "Rudy." All became superb bird dogs. Runner, whelped June 24, 2004, was a fine bird dog co-owned with Jessica Carlson. He had a spectacular performance pedigree with Ruffian's sire side, a line of five generations of males inducted into the Bird Dog Hall of Fame (HOF). They included National Field Champion (NFC) /DC Markar's Jac's A Dan D HOF, DC/AFC Jacque of Connie HOF, 2x NFC/ DC/ AFC Ban Dee HOF, and FC Kay-Cee Ban-Dee HOF. On his sire's dam's side was NAC/DC/ AFC Gringo De Britt HOF. On his dam's sire and dam's side were Ban Dee HOF, and Kay-Cee Ban Dee HOF, FC/AFC Scipio Spinks HOF, NFC/FC/ AFC Hi Proof Rum Runner HOF, NFC/FC/AFC Bean's Blaze HOF, and DC Scipio's Little Chick HOF.

Runner's impeccable pedigree and performance composed a complete package dog. He was a natural pointer and retrieved over water. As a puppy he ran with enthusiasm in the same way that his dam did. He was as consistent as

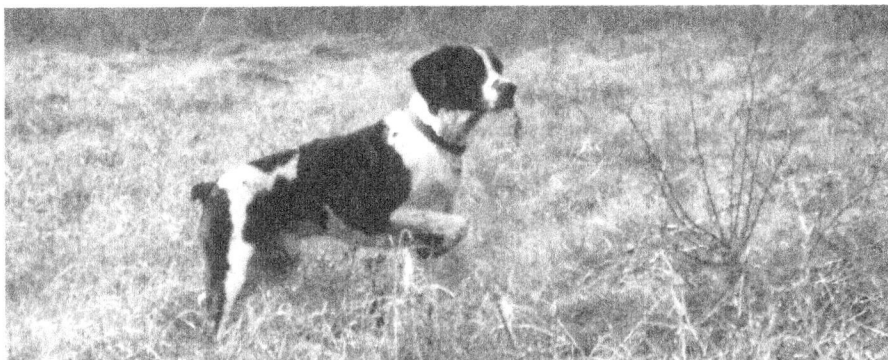

Ruffian on Bob White Quail pointing in Alabama.

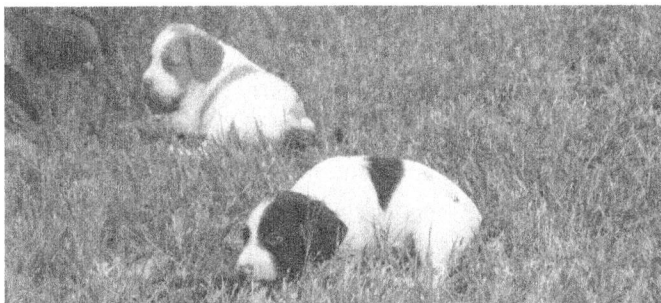

*Breton's Gold Run Runner (AKC SR18309201) "Runner,"
then 6 weeks old with littermate Page.*

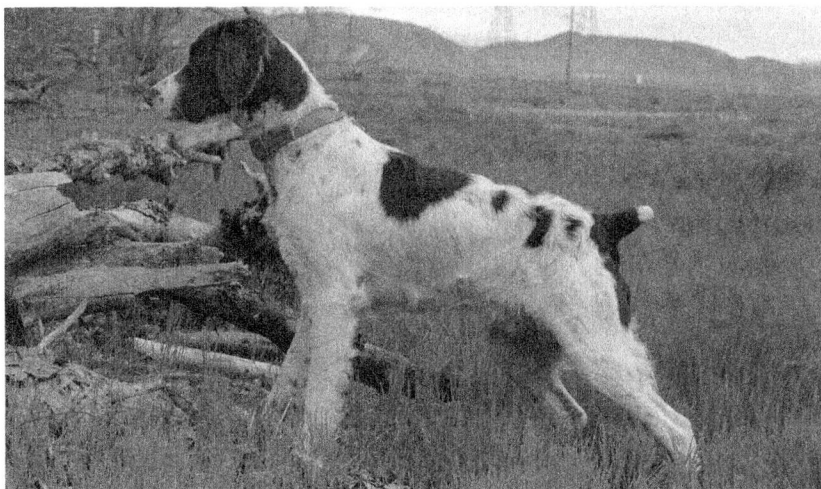

Runner on point Bob White Quail, Santa Nella, California, 18 months old.

253

Hank, who was runner-up in the All Age National Championship four times. Hank was tireless and, like Runner, never was flat. Runner at 8 months of age ran as big as an adult all-age dog with high caliber. What a joy to see this young dog run an unimaginable distance and to the front. On an occasion while running him as a juvenile derby dog in Eastern Washington, he ran far ahead and out of sight. I rode my horse, Blaze, to the front and a mile away, I found Runner standing on point, scenting a pheasant. What an amazing juvenile run, which unfortunately was not seen at the time under judgment.

As my age was advancing, I placed Runner with a well-known professional trainer and handler to break him as a finished adult dog. He finished him as a derby dog, along with puppy point accounts for 4 points toward championship. In the breaking process, he developed a diminishing desire to run, and avoided getting far from the trainer and handler. It became obvious that something had happened in training and I, according to field trial jargon, "pulled him" and brought him home.

I began to run him in training and he did well for me, but I was not able to show him often. After I brought Runner home he would soften on point and at times lie down as I approached him to put birds in the air. His reluctance was as pronounced as if I had placed a training electronic collar on him, but I never used voltage, only sound, after bringing him home. Most dogs like Runner develop manmade faults in training and care must be given to all dogs. I decided to place him with Scott and Linda Azevedo, second- and third-generation handlers and trainers at the famous Nelson Kennels in Los Banos, California. The Nelson training and handling facility was organized by a college-educated engineer, Norm Nelson. Norm taught his daughter Linda and grandson Scott to be honest, dedicated, devoted, and gentle in training. The Azevedos avoided causing bad habits or manmade faults in field dogs due to flawed training methods, particularly prohibiting use of an electronic jolting collar. Scott and Linda within a few months had Runner standing tall without softening on point. Runner again began to enjoy pointing and proudly holding point. Scott placed 20 field trial points on Runner toward field championship, in which only 10 points are required to earn FC. He did not have a 3-point major win in a American Brittany Club (ABC) local club sponsored trial needed to finish as an FC. He was retired at age 7 because of the AFC forced rule to attend a Brittany sponsored trial, which became few in number in the California circuit.

I continued to hunt with Runner at a hunt club. Even though he was a big running dog he enjoyed staying within a couple of hundred yards of me, and held point for many minutes until approached to place birds in the air. He continued to be a staunch pointer, holding after the bird was shot and given the command to fetch. If the bird was missed, he stood until released. While running he stops immediately if the bird flushes. He would be a FC if another breed, but the 3-point major win must be achieved in a Brittany sponsored trial. Runner is truly a complete hunting dog, a joy to hunt upland game.

Runner's littermate Page, co-owned with Christine Zink, was a pleasure to train and show in the field. She was a natural like Runner, a fine bird dog. Page ran in stakes referred to as gun dog stakes, meaning she was generally running and handling closer in than dogs like Tubby and Runner that ran in all age events. Chris and Bud Zink became friends almost immediately after I met them coming down the steps from the clubhouse at Hastings Island Hunting Preserve, where they had registered for Northern California Fun Days the end of July 2002. The resulting friendship involved the entire family on both sides. This is an example of the strong relationships that come through owning a dog

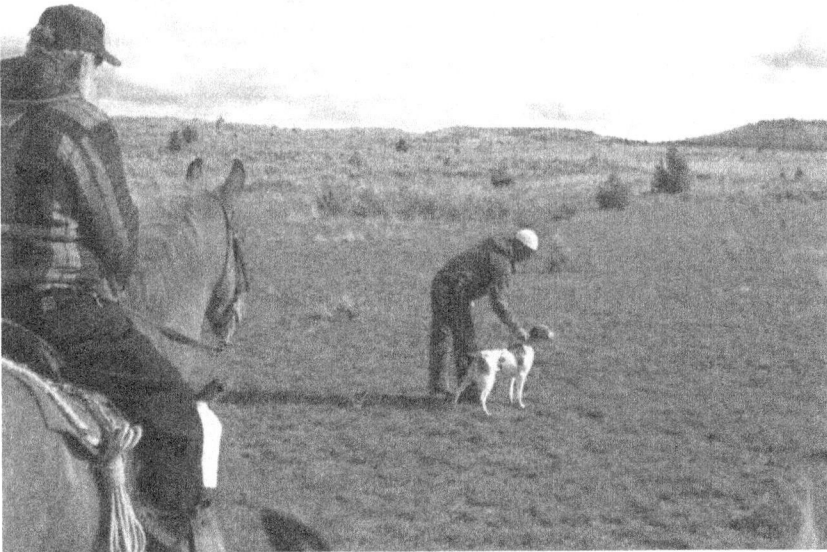

DC/AFC Breton's Truckee River Gold (AKC SR18309202), "Page," held by Paul Doiron at the Breakaway Western Futurity in Madras, Oregon, 2006.

and sharing the joys of canine-human bonds. Jessica Carlson finished Page as a DC in a short course of showing in one season. Page was closely bonded to Chris and Bud Zink and to members of our family. The co-ownership was a perfect arrangement.

"Rudy" was purchased by Mr. Jim McCann of Fairbanks, Alaska. This liver-and-white-colored male proved to be an outstanding upland game bird dog for several species of grouse. Jim wrote a book called *Upland Hunting in Alaska,* in which Rudy is mentioned and seen in a photograph. James McCann also owned two other dogs, Rusty and Charlie, from Breton Kennels.

Unplanned Mating: Captain and Tubby

Captain had an unplanned mating with DC/AFC Chikamin's Tub O'Gold. The resultant littermates were soft in training with a desire to run and find game. I became aware from this accidental mating that a soft dog mated to a bold dog such as Tubby results in softness. Most American Brittany owners have accepted Brittanys as genetically soft in various ways. This accepted trait can be changed if breeders want all-around bold dogs and try to eliminate softness. The softness trait is genetically dominant and should not be used when boldness is a breeding goal.

Breton's Heart of Gold, who Joe Bevier from Portland, Oregon, purchased, was a structurally fine-boned, small Brittany who was always ready to run like her dam. She had a heart of gold, as she was named, and had gazelle-like speed. She won the all-age Western Brittany Futurity by going and staying to the front, with the brace mate left way behind. Another female pup, Breton's Golden Surprise, went to the home of Rick and Mari-Ann Green, and was a good hunting dog and special pet. George Stern from Palo Alto, California, purchased an orange roan, "Rusty," who had the stamina of an outstanding all-age dog but was never companied in field completion under judgment. Rusty, however, later in his life was shown in conformation and awarded CH.

Chuck and Mary Lou Fisher in Klamath Falls, Oregon, purchased an orange roan female, "Maggie," a fine pheasant and quail hunting dog. Two went to Texas and turned out to be good hunting dogs. They originally were intended to be field trial dogs, but because of softness and their fine bone structure, they were resold to hunting homes.

Another breeding

We had decided to stop breeding following the disappointing experience with Slash, Rick and Mari-Ann's Green's wonderful pup that developed acute neurological epilepsy. Mr. Charles Gilpin called to ask if I had an interest in breeding his bitch Pepper to Sun. At that miraculous moment I agreed and the pups from this mating brought new dimension to bird dog genetics at Breton Kennels.

Charles and Helen Gilpin owned French Roast Pepper SH (AKC SR32089502), "Pepper." They had been owners of Brittanys since 1949. Mr. Rick Smith's kennel in Virginia was the breeder. Pepper was exactly what experienced hunters wanted as a bird dog. Pepper earned a Senior Hunter (SH) designation and points toward Master Hunter (MH) in hunt tests. She did not compete in trials.

I had been hospitalized at the beginning of April 2010 for three days due to severely reduced blood volume. I felt good enough by April 8 to supervise Sun's mating that day with Pepper. This mating was a miracle because only one copulatory tie occurred at the end of Pepper's estrus cycle, with whelping of five puppies. I mentioned to Charles when he came for Pepper that one tie near the end of estrus rarely produces a litter.

Sam competed in all breed trials by earning 29 AKC championship points. Sam is a fine complete field dog who does all tasks naturally. He never fails to hold point, retrieve to hand, swim if necessary to bring back the game, and honor with extreme style. He has a loving personality, excels in wanting to please, and has added as littermates to the exceptional Breton Kennels gene pool. Sam is a seventh-generation roan-colored Brittany selected from the first in our line, Gianoli's Pat. In July 2016 Sam completed dual championship. He never had showed before May, and two months later he finished as a champion. He is a fine bird dog, shows extreme intensity on point, and loves to retrieve.

Dr. Jim and Mary Cullor selected Cookie, who at 3 years of age achieved FC and did well in the 2013 Brittany Gun Dog Nationals in Ionia Michigan, with honorable mention. Cookie is a superb bird dog who pointed and honored even before she was weaned. This exceptional ability was evident in field trials. She was awesome with a bold attitude in hunting and trialing. During the summer of 2015 Cookie was handled by Jessica Carlson in conformation AKC sponsored events. In a few weeks she achieved Dual Championship

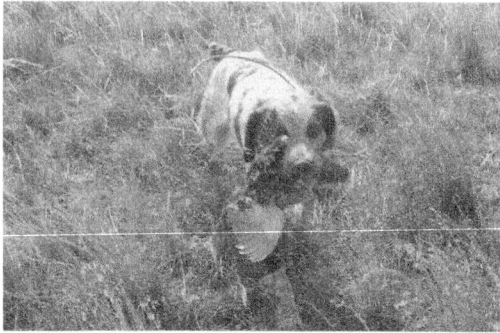

DC/FC Breton's Sam I Am (AKC SR5731604), " Sam,"
retrieving a sharp tail grouse in Montana, 2015.

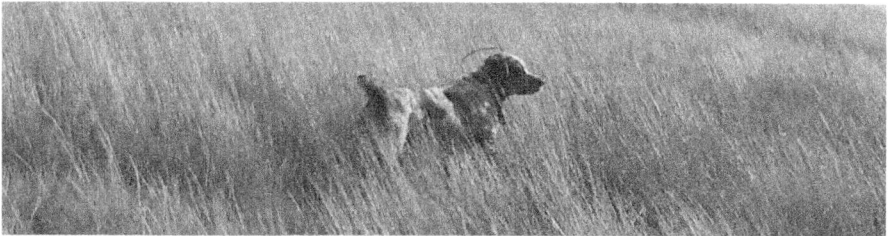

Sam pointing Hungarian partridge in Montana, 2015 (Compliments of Kyle Tetlow).

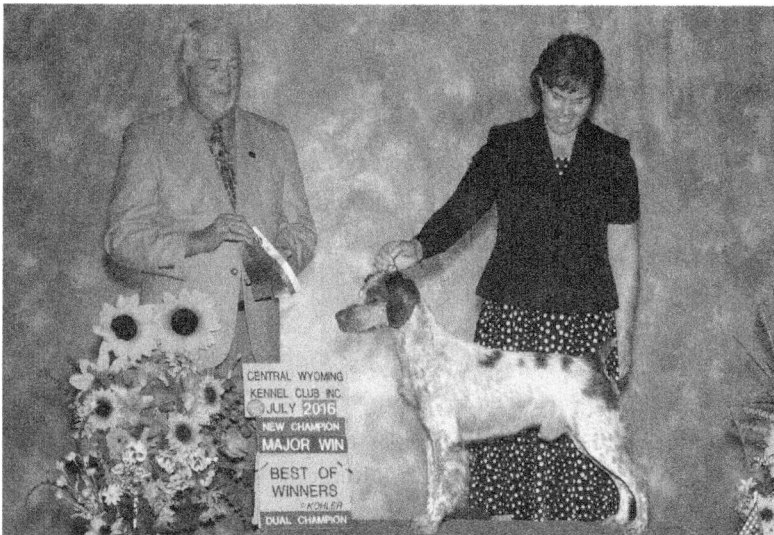

Sam as dual championship in Wyoming with Jessica Carlson, 2016.

(DC) on the Midwest show circuit. She continued to show after earning DC. A month later she finished as the third Brittany bitch to achieve Grand Champion and the first roan bitch to achieve such a high show honor. She added to the special genetic makeup of dogs bred at Breton Kennels. Her dam has added a special genetic input to the Breton Kennels gene pool.

Frannie, co-owned by Helen and Charles Gilpin, is intensely interested in hunting and always starts with extreme enthusiasm for her length of time in the field. Frannie is a good pointer and backs with style. She is a talented dog with wonderful conformation and runs with an effortless stride. She is a watchdog and barks when a stranger is on the property. She loves people and is kind with dogs. Linda and Scott Azevedo trained her for trials in the summer and fall of 2015. She impressed them and quickly advanced to being "steady to wing and shot" – meaning that she remained on point through the flush of the bird and the gunshot, until her handler commanded her to retrieve the fallen bird.

She was entered in Open Gun Dog and Open Limited Gun Dog categories at the NCBC trial at Hastings Island, August 15–16, 2015. On Saturday of the competition, she ran in AKC competition for the first time in the Open Gun Dog stake and placed second among 17 dogs entered. She had four steady

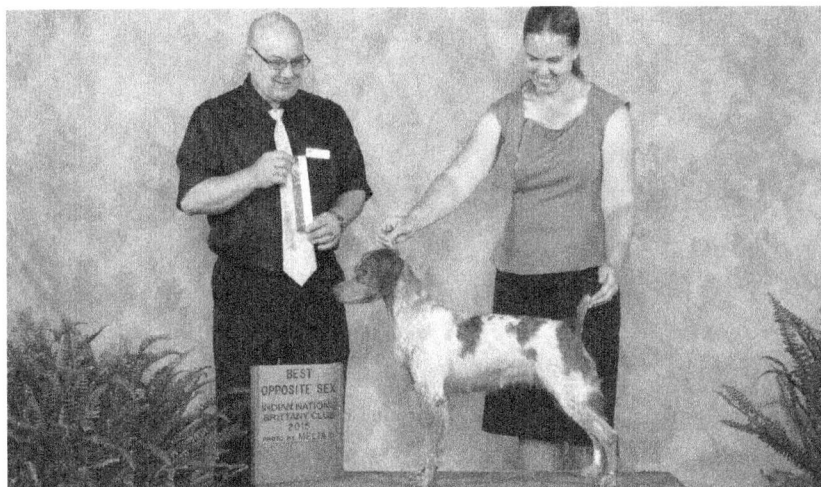

GC/FC Breton's Golden Heart of Pepper-Sun (AKC SR57131601), "Cookie."
Winner of Best of Opposite award at the Indian Nations Brittany Club in
Oklahoma, with Jessica Carlson showing, 2015.

finds. The 100-degree temperature that day did not prevent her from running with extreme enthusiasm. Frannie was called back after all braces were run to show the judges she could retrieve a shot bird. On Sunday she again had four finds that she handled perfectly. She ran with extreme enthusiasm even though the temperature hit 110 degrees. This was not a retrieving stake, so there was no call back to retrieve. She was awarded a blue ribbon in a 15-dog entry. This win entitled her to a needed 3-point major win in an American Brittany Club sponsored trial to be in line for AKC field championship. In the next trial she was entered, she was first in Open Limited Gun Dog and third in Open Gun Dog. This short history of Breton Kennels highlights our desire to improve the special Brittany breed. The Boy with the Wounded Thumb's closeness to dogs began as an infant living in rural Minnesota in the late 1920s associating with one special dog, a German shepherd named Rex.

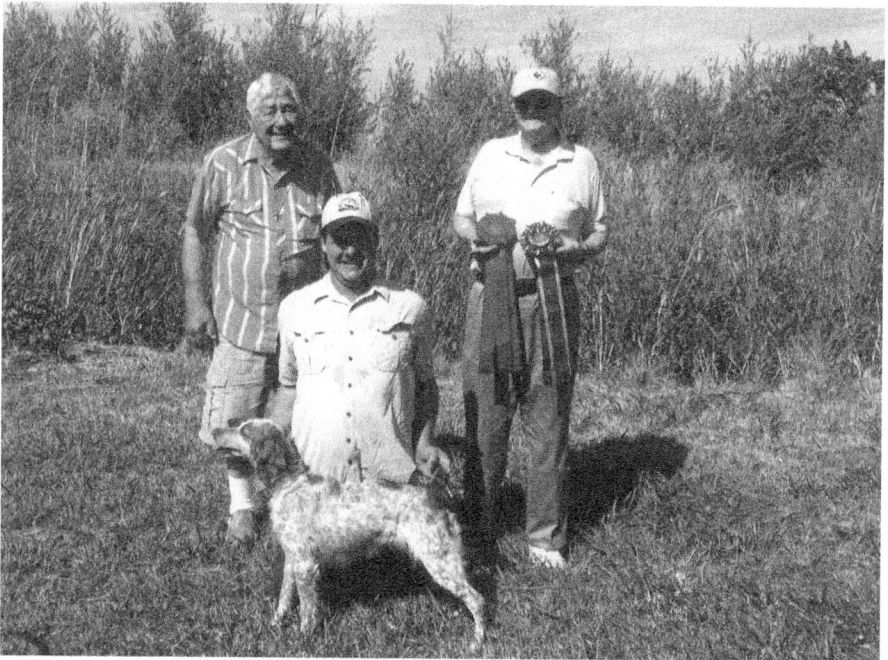

Breton's Frangelica A Toast to Pepper and Sam (AKC SR5731603), "Frannie" in August 2015 at Hastings Island in Dixon, California. At the time she was 6 years of age, and this was her first adult stakes in trialing winner in the Open Limited Gun Dog category and runner up in the Open Gun Dog competition. At left is Gordon Theilen, and at right are co-owner Charles Gilpin and handler Scott Azevido.

ABOUT THE AUTHOR

Gordon Theilen, DVM, ACVIM—Oncology, is one among a handful of internationally renowned veterinary comparative scientists who founded the discipline of veterinary oncology in the 1960s. He coauthored the first comprehensive veterinary oncology reference texts, *Veterinary Cancer Medicine*. The first volume was translated into Japanese. Noted for his stubborn refusal to concede to the ravages of cancer in animals, Dr. Theilen provided comprehensive information helping conquer neoplastic diseases in humans. He was a leader in combination cancer treatment, including chemotherapy, radiotherapy, and immunotherapy.

A professor at the University of California, Davis, School of Veterinary Medicine for 37 years, Dr. Theilen did basic research on cancer-causing viruses in horses, turkeys, cows, cats, and primates. In 1965 he identified and named stem cell sarcoma in turkeys, Reticuloendotheliosis. In 1969, he co-discovered Synder-Theilen Feline Sarcoma Virus (ST-FeSV), and he discovered the first and only Simian Sarcoma Virus, SSV-1 (WMSV), in 1971. This discovery led to recognition on the cover of Cancer Research, volume 42, August 1982, a journal of the American Association for Cancer Research.

In 1964-65, Dr. Theilen served a fellowship at the National Cancer Institute, Bethesda, Maryland, in the laboratory of Ray C. Bryan, and in 1972-73 he was a fellow at the Royal Marsden Hospital, Chester Beatty Institute in London. In 1979-80 he was an Alexander von Humboldt Research Institute senior scientist at the School of Medicine's Department of Virology, Justus Liebig University, Giessen, Germany. He also worked in veterinary pathology there. He visited other countries to help veterinarians and physicians understand cancer-causing retroviral infections. He was honored to give the annual pathology lecture for the schools of medicine and veterinary medicine at the University of Edinburgh. Theilen waged a one-medicine war on cancer, and was honored by UC Davis on his 80th birthday with the Theilen Tribute Symposium in recognition of 50 years of cancer research. Scientific papers were presented by leading cancer researchers.

His students – interns, residents, fellows and postdocs – have spanned the world with their influence and leadership affecting many other related areas of veterinary and human comparative medicine.

Dr. Theilen was awarded University of California, Davis, School of Veterinary Medicine outstanding Alumni Achievement Award in 1987. He was active in several professional associations appointed Honor Roll Member of the American Associations of Veterinary Medicine, in 1999. A charter member of the Veterinary Cancer Society and, Charter Member of American College of Internal Medicine-Oncology. He helped organize, and was a charter member of the International Association for Comparative Research on Leukemia and Related Diseases (ACRLRD) in 1962, and served as a world committee member from 1969 to 1974. He served on Scientific Review Committee of Leukemia and Lymphoma Society in America from 1970 to 1975. He chaired the Annual Scientific and Membership Meeting in San Francisco in 1973. He was a member of the WHO Committee, Staging Tumors in Animals from 1972 to 1978, which consisted of five other international leaders. He has been a member of American Association for Cancer Research since 1960, the Society of Phi Zeta since 1958, and the Society of Sigma Xi since 1960.

Dr. Theilen has been active for nearly 50 years in the American Kennel Club – breeding, training, and showing champion field trial Brittanys. His dogs gained over 100 AKC field placements with 50 percent first place, 25 percent second place, and third and fourth place 15 percent each. Three of his dogs were dual champions, 12 field champions, and three amateur field champions. He collected genetic samples from Brittanys during field trials over many years. His breeding programs have improved genetic abilities as outstanding bird dogs. He was named to the American Field Bird Dog Field Trial Hall of Fame in 2006, recognized in 2007 in the Brittany Hall of Fame, and honored for his service as a consultant and board member for the American Brittany Club from 1985 to 1990. He was nominated a life member in Northern California Brittany Club.

CPSIA information can be obtained
at www.ICGtesting.com
Printed in the USA
BVOW06s1002050217
475333BV00014B/1017/P

9 781937 317300